The Teenage Social Media Detox

7 Simple Steps on How Teens Unplugged in the Digital World

E. T. Mulloney

Contents

To Patrick, my ever-loving and steadfast spouse, you are the bedrock of my life, next only to God Himself.

This book is a heartfelt dedication to you, the constant wellspring of love, encouragement, and inspiration in my journey. With your presence, each page of our shared story becomes a beautiful and meaningful part of our life together as a family, and our cherished fur companion, Tiggy boy, is an essential character in this adventure. We are beyond blessed!

Introduction

The life of a teenager dates back to the beginning of humanity. On the other hand, social media is a relatively newer concept. What was once a science fiction idea to some has now become an extension of our personalities. Of course, teenagers from hundreds of years ago didn't have electricity, let alone access to the internet. However, a teenager just 15 years ago might've had limited time on the computer, having to share it with other siblings or whoever wanted to use the phone.

The times have rapidly changed, and now we can pull up anything we want to see at the tip of our fingertips so long as our phones are charged and we have service. Even when we don't have access to the internet, we can play games, communicate with friends, and take pictures with just a few taps and clicks.

All of the noises, sights, and options become ingratiated into every aspect of our lives, altering our thoughts, behaviors, and emotions. In a way, this is a good thing, as we have access to information and communication like never before. But when use becomes mismanaged, it can be overstimulating, frustrating, and addictive.

Teenagers and young adults today are the first to experience life in the presence of social media throughout their most developmental years. From social networking forums to business pages that could impact your career, social media is an enigma that is constantly changing history.

Navigating this is challenging for any age, but the more innovations we see, the more reliant we are on the internet as a whole. Video streaming services are replacing cable, texts are replacing letters, and emails are replacing paper mail. All of this is happening on a daily basis.

In one study, it was found that 95% of teens between the ages of 13–17 have used YouTube, with 77% of them using it daily (Gelles-Watnick & Vogels, 2023). Life with easy access to the internet can be very impactful to your health, especially during a time when your mind and body are still developing.

Research also shows that the older the teen, the more likely they are to state they use the internet almost constantly (Massarat, 2022). What this shows is that our accessibility and use might increase over time. The more often we repeat a pattern, the more likely it is to become a part of our daily life. Some teens report using social media for up to nine hours daily ("Social Media," 2018).

If you feel pressured and stressed by school and family to reduce your digital usage, you're not alone. This is a common issue for teens, but that is why it's even more important for youth to work on their time and health management. If you can learn the skills to be mindful as early as possible, you can break free from the habit of overusing social media.

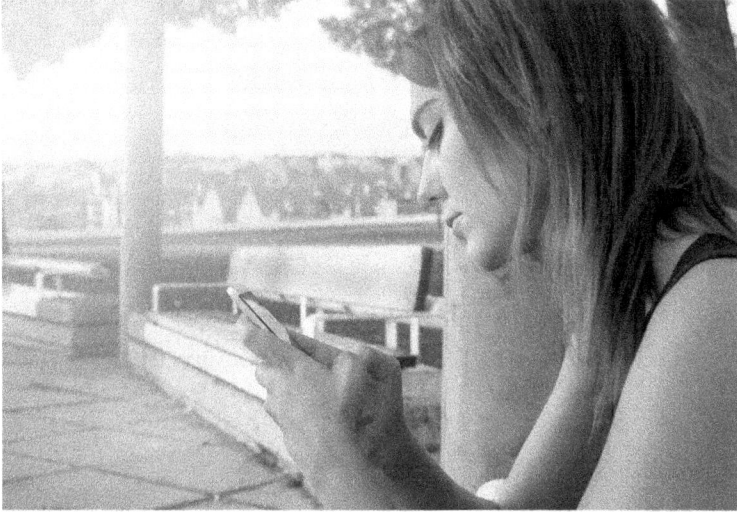

Social media use is time-consuming and keeps us distracted from things we might rather be doing. It creates a sense of urgency within us that can influence our anxiety levels. It changes our thoughts which will eventually start to change how we view life itself. Most of us feel the effects of excessive social media use, but knowing how to realistically reduce it can be a challenge in itself.

There are many benefits of going through a detox that you can't comprehend until you are experiencing the process because of the hold it has over your thoughts and actions. The relief and stress reduction you will feel will help you realize just how invaluable excessive social media use can be.

Not all social media is a bad thing, though! There's a reason that we are so enthralled and entertained by these innovations. There are endless ways to connect and consume information, but enjoying the benefits of social media can be challenging when we don't have mindfulness over our habits.

By becoming more aware of our habits, taking steps to reduce usage, and finding new ways to flourish in our lives, we can take back power over these habits to build a positively impactful relationship with our phones.

Social media use is very impactful on a developing mind, so it's important to implement methods of reducing screen time for all ages, but especially teenagers. There is so much life to be enjoyed in youth, and getting consumed by the pressures of social media can make it difficult to take advantage of.

The dependency on social media is frustrating and time-consuming. It holds a power over us that can make us feel trapped by our urges to check in with what's happening on the internet. It doesn't have to be this way, however, so taking the next steps to reduce your social media use will help you declutter your mind for increased emotional management.

How to Use This Book

The readings in this book will travel between seven essential steps as seen through the seven chapters. Each one can be done in a step-by-step process, but take it at your own pace and make adjustments to the process as you see fit. The relationship we all have with our phones is an individual one, and it's not easy to transform it for the better.

The seven steps will provide guidance and practical, applicable steps to reduce the use of social media and experience the benefits of controlling this habit. When initiative is taken to reduce stress and improve the quality of life, it will make it a substantial and long-lasting trait not just for your teen years, but for your life as an adult as well.

You will find tips for reducing social media use alongside methods to replace the time spent on the internet with more productive habits. It's suggested to use a journal, notebook, or digital document to track progress and write down notes and reflections.

A Note to Parents

Many readers are likely teens themselves, but it's important for parents of adolescents alike to consider their and their child's social media use. Much of what a teenager learns is through what is seen by them. If you are a parent who struggles with social media use, your teen might be getting their habits from you. This means the tips and methods used don't only work for adolescents! By implementing healthier habits into your life as a parent, you will be able to help your child make improvements as well.

Regardless of your age, reducing social media use is *always* a good thing. Knowing the ins and outs of internet management will empower you to maintain healthy and productive habits so you can find success in whatever your goals may be.

1. Understand the Impact

Social media has become such an ingrained part of our habitual nature that it's hard to comprehend just how detrimental it's been to our lives. The use of our phones is such a passive activity that we don't even realize we're on it sometimes.

"Passive" refers to the way that we might unknowingly participate in a habit. "Active," conversely, is something that requires a bit more of our attention. For example, tapping your foot or biting your nails is something that happens a bit more passively. You might unknowingly chew on your pencil or twirl your hair. Painting your nails, using your pencil, or stretching your foot is a bit more active.

Our phone use has become second nature. Have you ever found yourself lifting up your phone and scrolling through social media without even thinking about it? Every time you leave the house, your phone might be the first thing to check and ensure you have before heading out the door. At least if you forget your keys, you can call someone to let you in!

Of course, not all phone use is bad. And not all social media is bad. We can protect ourselves and stay safe through phone use, for one. A problem arises when we lose track of just how much time is spent online, though. This time could be spent doing other things, like studying or socializing. Too much phone use is associated with a decrease in mental health. In fact, teens who are using social media for three or more hours a day are more likely to experience mental health problems (Miller, 2022).

The first step in overcoming social media use is understanding the impact that social media has had on your mind.

Why is social media so addictive? Why is it so hard to just ignore the internet on your own? What makes it so enticing to want to constantly and habitually check in with the online world?

The first step to take to reduce your screen time use is to utilize methods of noticing screen time habits and become more aware of how you are using your devices so that your usage of them becomes more of an active habit rather than a passive one.

The Addictive Nature

Using a phone can produce dopamine, so we literally become addicted to using it (Goldman, 2021). In addition, research has shown that those who depend on social media use can exhibit symptoms similar to substance abuse ("Are You Addicted," n.d.).

First and foremost, phones keep us connected. That's what they were made for! Over 100 years ago, we wanted to be able to talk to people who were not in the same physical space that we were. We wanted to be able to communicate emergencies and stay in touch with people. We wanted to be able to relay important information and provide many different services to individuals.

Nowadays, we need phones to survive.

You need to call different services when you need help or have issues. You need to call your doctor to make an appointment. You need to call 911 in the case of extreme emergencies. You need to call your school to let them know that you might not be in attendance that day.

There are so many small ways of communication that we still depend on our phones for. In addition to that, the use of a phone has become incredibly twisted and reshaped over time. Nowadays, we use phones mostly to entertain ourselves. We entertain ourselves by talking and chatting with friends. We entertain ourselves by watching funny videos or looking at what our friends are currently up to. We check in with stories of strangers and celebrities, and we also express ourselves through social media. We share our own thoughts online, and all of this helps us to stay more connected to other people.

Who would have thought that in 1876, when the phone was first invented, they would have become what they are today?

Not only do we stay connected to friends, peers, and other important officials, but we also stay connected to the world. That is more true now than ever before and it is always going to be more true the further along we get in technology.

You used to have to rely on letters to connect with someone across the world. Now, you can video chat with them or watch their live posts on social media. You can figure out what is happening at the furthest point away from you in the universe by checking in online.

This makes us feel more informed. It makes us feel more like we are a part of our world.

What we haven't realized, however, especially as teenagers, is that this different type of connection can also make us feel really disconnected.

Social media can elicit many feelings of isolation. You might see a group of people hanging out online and feel as though you don't have as many friends as they do. You might focus all of your time and energy on the internet and spend your free time in the digital world, therefore neglecting real social circles in the physical world.

Our phones help us see what other people are up to and they provide instant news updates, making this a vital part of our lives. When we're disconnected from the internet, it can make us feel as though we're disconnected from our reality.

The urge and desire to be a part of something bigger is a natural emotion that humans have evolved to have throughout time. Different animals have different survival instincts. Just think of the way a mouse habitates, eats, and lives in general compared to a spider. As humans, we prefer social settings and to be a part of a group. Think of primates in the wild and how they are seen in groups, versus a wolf, who might be seen as more of a loner animal. We rely on protection and unity to help us survive and thrive.

Thousands of years ago, we formed groups that consisted of hunters and gatherers. Some people were better at trekking out in the world and fighting and killing animals. Others were better at foraging.

The mix of different groups helped people develop the cognitive and survival skills that we have, which have made us one of the most advanced species on the planet.

This level of advancement has maintained many natural social urges within us in modern times. We want to be a part of a group. We want to be recognized and acknowledged by other people. We want others to see that we are special and unique so that they see value in us. If we don't feel valued, then it can make us feel really isolated and like we're not an important part of society.

Recognizing this natural human urge can help you understand why it feels so good to be connected, not just in your social circle, but in the world in general. This natural human instinct is also why it can be so addictive to use your phone.

In addition, we are also highly addicted to our cell phones because they are so accessible.

You can't go out to eat and party with your friends every single night. You can't go to the movies every night. You can't go to a comedy show, zoo, or other place of entertainment day after day. Whether your parents say that you're not allowed to do that or you just don't have it in your budget, it's not realistic for us to be hanging out with our friends or doing fun activities every day of the week. What we can do, however, is check in with our friends every day, multiple times a day online.

Our phones are also extremely accessible because they're small and mobile. Even just as recently as a decade ago, not everybody had a cell phone, and they likely had to share phone use or data with other people.

Two to three decades ago, the average person didn't have a cell phone at all.

If you did, it might have been a luxury in the family. You also likely had to share internet usage with other people. In the days of landlines, only one person could use either the phone or the computer at a time, so you had a very limited amount of time to spend online and scroll through social media.

Nowadays, everybody has not only their phones but other devices like tablets and laptops that help keep them connected to other people. We also have many types of gaming systems and online video games that we connect to our friends with.

In more recent years, we have developed many different types of video chatting software, allowing us to hang out with other people from the comfort of our own homes without everybody having to meet up in a physical group. This accessibility makes it even more enticing to want to sit on your phone or other devices and spend time in the digital world. There is also plenty of variety, so you can do all of these things in just one sitting.

Phones fit into our pockets, purses, and small bags, and smartwatches even allow us to have notifications and messages strapped to our bodies at all times.

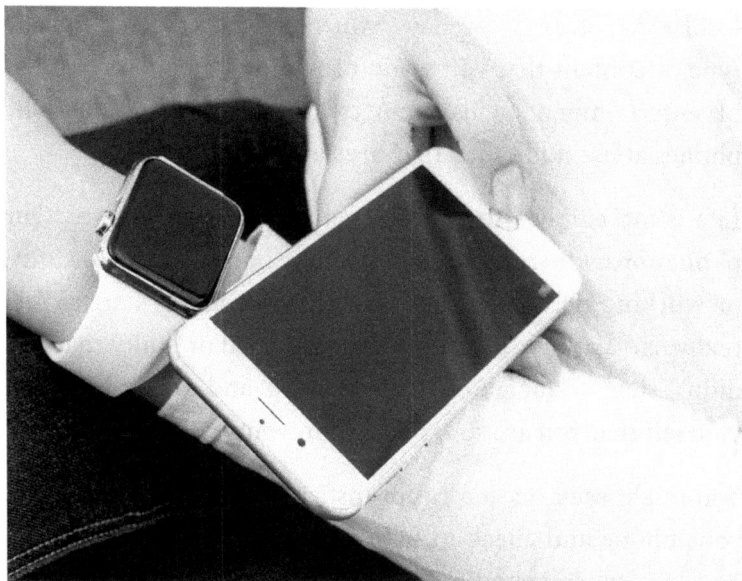

The addictive nature of phones exists because of how purely accessible they are. Consider anybody who is struggling with an addiction, whether they can't seem to give up sweets, or they're dependent on alcohol. Sometimes these things are not as easily accessible, therefore, it's easier to avoid that addiction. For example, if you're underage, you can't buy alcohol. If you don't have any money, you can buy those sweets. It's a lot harder to get access to some of these more addictive substances. However, if you have a cell phone and access to the internet, you can use it as much as you'd like.

Our phones also give us access to information all across the world. We can explore things that we never could have without technology. You can learn about interesting facts. You can watch movies and listen to music made by people across the world. You used to have to rely on whatever was on cable TV at night, or whatever you could purchase at your local video store. Nowadays, you can Google search for any type of content that you want, providing an endless amount of entertainment. This connects to the next reason why phones are so addicting: they are also very distracting.

Life is incredibly stressful, no matter what age you are. Our phones provide instant relief. If you're bored, trying to study, or working on a paper late at night, you might start to feel really bad about yourself. You feel ashamed or guilty that you didn't start sooner. You feel annoyed and frustrated with yourself that you are so far behind in your work.

You might seek out a form of instant relief. You can pick up your phone and check in with what your friends are doing. You can text somebody and complain about how much work you have to do. You can pull up funny videos on TikTok and scroll endlessly, distracting yourself from the stress of life.

This is also ingrained in our psychology. We want to find immediate relief when we feel bad. If you're hot, you might turn a fan on. If you're cold, you might put a jacket on. If you're hungry, you could eat a snack. If you're tired, you go to bed.

If you're unhappy, you find something to make you feel good.

Your phone is accessible and it's always around, so you always have something that is going to make you feel good. Anything that provides you with happiness or joy is something that your brain is going to log and remember for the future.

Next time you're feeling sad, your brain thinks to itself, *Oh, my phone makes me feel good. I'll check in on social media. I'll watch that one person's story on Instagram. I'll see what everybody is up to on Tiktok. I'll check if any of my subscriptions have posted a new video on YouTube. I'll see if there are any good deals on the food delivery app.*

Your brain associates all these good things with instant relief from your stress. Since we are dealing with stress multiple times a day, we are seeking that happiness through our phones multiple times a day as well.

Phones are there when we're bored with schoolwork or panicking about something else in our personal life. They become our best friends and biggest support systems without us realizing that they are also hurting us at the same time.

Our phones also allow us to even Google symptoms of the negative things that we're feeling. If you're stressed or anxious, you might be dealing with a rapid heartbeat or perhaps are starting to sweat. Maybe you Google signs of a heart attack thinking that your rapid heartbeat is a sign that you're physically in danger. You might have trouble breathing so you start looking up what it means to have symptoms of shortness of breath.

You can see if there is an instant answer or immediate relief from some of the things that are stressing you out and making you feel panicked. However, once you open up Google, you might close out of it, and then instinctually open up another app, distracting yourself even further.

In addition to all of these reasons that phones are so addictive, we also have to remember that *they are designed to make us feel good.*

Some apps are designed to be addictive. Think about endless scrolling. Many apps allow you to keep scrolling forever, constantly providing you with a fresh news feed. This makes it incredibly enticing because, even when you notice that you've spent an hour scrolling through Instagram, you might simply swipe up again only to see many new posts from your friends.

By the time you finish watching all of your friends' stories, more have been posted, therefore creating an endless cycle of constantly streaming content.

Phones are meant to be user-friendly. They are designed so that anybody can use them whether you're 13 or 93. They are supposed to be intuitive, so they are designed to naturally align with some of your physical and mental habits. They are colorful, they make fun noises, and they are enjoyable to use, even when you're just doing something like typing. Think about the little sounds that the clicks make or how you can incorporate emojis into what you're texting. All of this is specifically crafted so that you find more enjoyment from your experience using a phone.

We can customize the sound of our notifications so that when you hear a certain friend text you, you hear that exciting noise, making it more likely that you're going to keep scrolling online.

Like anything that makes us feel good, our brains are going to want to use this as much as possible, not just when we are seeking relief from stress. They become habitual and second nature, so before you know it, you become fully addicted to this habit.

On top of that, we *have* to use our phones. We have to check emails, check our bank accounts, and even do our homework on the internet. There's so much reliance on the World Wide Web that even when you want to escape it, you can't.

How can you tell if you are addicted to your phone? One thing to start noticing is how often you think about using social media, even when you're not using it. Do you have the urge to check in even when you can't? Do you find yourself sitting in class, wanting to pull out your phone even though it's against school policy? Do you plan and think out texts and emails when you're doing simple things like showering or brushing your teeth?

Do you find yourself constantly checking your phone even when you're hanging out and socializing with other people? Do you find that you are on your phone more often than you are enjoying hobbies, like different sports or creative activities?

As we start to unravel all of the intricacies and small details of the ways that we are connected to our phones, we can begin to improve this habit.

It's also important to note that your algorithm is set to specify what you want to look at, making it even more addicting. What your news feed looks like on different apps is going to be completely different from the person sitting next to you, even if the two of you have similar tastes and interests. There are specific formulas created to gather our personal information and use that against us so that we want to keep scrolling, make purchases, and stay connected online.

For some, this is a good thing. It means that you filter out the things that you're not interested in and can provide you with things that you actually care about. However, it can be incredibly harmful because you unknowingly get fed misinformation, hatred online, and other things that are meant to entice you and keep your attention.

When we are not conscious of our social media use and how impactful it can be to our lives, we end up becoming so addicted that it becomes a habit that feels impossible to break.

Identifying Screentime Habits

It's estimated that at least 10% of the population has a social media addiction in the US alone (Quinn, 2023). This number is even higher for teens, and it's hard to tell how great it really could be since many people are unknowingly dependent on their phones.

80% of teens believe social media makes them feel more connected to their friends (Anderson et al., 2022). When we see social media use as a good thing, though, it's hard to maintain control over it. While it's true that it does have some benefits, we still must be aware and conscious of how it is impacting our lives so that we can stay one step ahead of our use. When you do this, you allow yourself to actually enjoy the benefits while reducing the negative side effects.

It's hard to keep track of how much social media use you're participating in on a daily basis because we aren't always taught that it's something that we're supposed to track. When it comes to other addictive habits like eating, you're told that you're supposed to monitor how much food you're eating in a day. You should pay attention to how many candy bars, bags of chips, sodas, and other potentially unhealthy snacks you're consuming. When it comes to social media, there's no set limit. We're not provided with a guideline of how much social media we should be using. Of course, some people might recommend not using it at all, but for many, we understand that this is an unrealistic precedent to set.

In addition, social media use is not illegal and has actually been actively encouraged within our society. Everywhere you look, you'll see ads telling you to check something out online. Every business you go to has a little symbol or sign next to their social media tags so that you can easily look them up and follow them. When you meet new people, they ask for your social media so that they can stay connected with you when the two of you are not together.

Because of this, it's very hard to monitor just how much we're using it. As a teen, it's also difficult to stay focused on the amount of social media that you use because your brain is still developing. You are still dealing with impulse control, and that's a hard thing to manage on your own.

Parents can sometimes monitor how much social media we use, but it's very easy to get around some of those rules and restrictions, especially when they are not around constantly.

It's up to you to be proactive and to take initiative in reducing your screentime habits. The first step is to keep track of how much social media you're using so that you can get a better gauge of the way this habit is intertwined with your daily life. Start by using phone tracking software. If you have an iPhone, this is a feature that's already built into your phone and is also an easily accessible app on many other types of devices. This will keep track of how frequently you use different social media apps. It will give you a breakdown, and some apps also help you track progress between days and weeks.

It's also important after you start tracking your phone use to notice any trends. Did you notice that maybe on Sunday you spent six hours online whereas on Monday and Tuesday, you only spent about an hour each? Perhaps you were busier with other things happening on those days. Now you know that next week when Sunday comes around, it's better to have a plan for what to do that day to keep you distracted so that you are less likely to spend all of it scrolling the internet. Did you find that maybe one day you used a lot of social media after you had a particularly hard or stressful day?

Is there something that you enjoy doing that allows you to not check in with your phone at all? Whatever keeps you away from your phone is something to add more of into your life, and whatever makes you want to use your phone at an excessive level is something to monitor and reduce. Noticing these small trends and habits of your social media use will make you more aware of how you've been utilizing that habit so that you can monitor it in the future.

After you start tracking some of the social media time that you spend online, write it down in a notebook. Keep a separate record of it so that you can reinforce just how much time you've been spending online. It's easy to open your phone tracking app and see that you spent three hours on Instagram yesterday, but what you can also do is swipe away and not check in with that. However, saying "I spent three hours on Instagram yesterday," and writing it down in your journal, makes you go back over that idea again so that you can fully grasp just how much time was spent on the internet.

After you start keeping better track of your habits, it's important to set limits for how many minutes you can use certain apps a day. Use third-party apps or the built-in feature on your devices to set time limits.

This means giving each app a 15-minute daily time limit, or perhaps 30 minutes. If you only use one or two social media apps, try to keep social media use under an hour each day. That might sound hard to do, but what you will discover is that you can get just as much from social media within the hour as you might get when you are spending three hours or more on it a day.

These app limits also help you gain a better awareness of checking in on your phone without even realizing you're doing it. It gives you kind of a stop sign before you fall into the trap of endless scrolling. For example, if you use up your 15-minute time limit on Instagram, you might click Instagram on your phone, open it, and get prompted with a reminder that you've already reached your time limit for that day. It's a small reminder that helps you close your phone and put your focus elsewhere.

The last part of raising more awareness over your phone use is to go through notifications. There is no reason to have notifications for social media whatsoever. Unless you are a social media manager or that is part of your career, you do not need constant and instant updates from social media. The only notifications you should have on are for text messages or phone calls from specific people. This would include your parents, partner, or maybe some close friends. You can have notifications to get texts from a grandparent, a teacher, or somebody else whom you have to check in with. Other than that, silence group chats and turn off notifications for things like Instagram, Reddit, TikTok, Snapchat, and other social media that you might be using.

Our brains can actually start to associate phone notifications with "pleasurable feelings," conditioning us to feel a sense of urgency or excitement when one goes off ("Constant Smartphone Notifications," 2022).

You can set specific times to check in with these apps throughout the day, therefore allowing you to check in with all of your notifications at once. You can check in daily so you still stay up to date with friends, but you don't have to check it the second that you receive a notification. Is it important to respond to a meme that a friend sent you? Do you have to watch that video that your partner just sent you? Chances are you don't. The constant notifications that we get are little reminders throughout the day to grab our phone and start checking in.

Imagine if the snacks from the cupboard called your name. Imagine if all of the ice cream in your freezer made a little dinging noise throughout the day! You would be snacking on things much more often than you should.

Checking in on social media does not have to be an all-day, frequent thing. You can set aside specific time periods to stay connected with the world around you. Notifications are incredibly distracting and can pull your focus throughout the day. Even if you don't attend to that notification right away, you might start thinking about it.

For example, if you're in the shower and you hear five text messages go off in a row, you might start panicking, wondering if you should cut your shower short so that you can attend to those notifications. When you get out, you realize that it's just your friends sending GIFs and memes. Notifications create a false sense of urgency and stress when we constantly hear them.

It's up to you to go back through and identify the emotions, responses, and habits that you have as a result of social media use. There's a reason that you're here, reading this book, and seeking help. Chances are, you've already identified the ways social media has had a negative impact on your life.

List these things out. For example, you might write down the following:

- I feel anxious after spending too much time on TikTok.
- I feel tired and bored after a long day of social media use.

Once you're able to label your feelings and emotions connected to social media, it gives you greater insight into the habits that have been destructive in your life. This period of enlightenment is crucial for putting your social media addiction at bay.

Reminders

- **Step #1**: Understand the impact that social media can have on one's life.

Most of us already know that social media can be addictive—that's why we're here in the first place. But knowing the inner workings of that addictive nature is important so that we can come up with strategies to reduce screen time and take back power over our lives. Not only is excessive social media use unhealthy, but it can also be potentially dangerous.

2. Know the Dangers

S ocial media doesn't damage the body in the way that other addictions do, like drugs and sugar, so it's easy to assume it's not that dangerous. However, the long-term effects are certainly something to be concerned about. There are endless warnings given to teens about drunk driving or doing drugs and the severity behind these is scary, as the worst-case scenario is often death or injury. Social media is something more subtle and takes longer to show signs of overuse. You don't always get addicted to it overnight. While social media can lead to death or harm by breaking down our mental health, there aren't as many instant physical side effects, so it can be more difficult to pinpoint just how damaging it can be.

Social media use can impact our health and increase anxiety. Noticing the symptoms we've been dealing with will make it easier to reduce usage overall.

The Risks of Being Online

Your digital footprint will never be erased ("Understanding Your Digital Footprint," 2019). You can delete social media apps, change your username, and shut off your internet altogether, but remnants of your online activity will always linger on the World Wide Web.

Social media is all about sharing bits and pieces of your life online. Most of us consent to some of our personal information being shared with the world. We willingly post what we ate for dinner. We willingly share selfies. We consent to allow people to look at this content. However, there is so much that we don't understand about our privacy.

Whenever prompted with a text box that says "accept here," it's easy to click the checkmark and move on to the next stage. When you're asked, "Do you consent?", you might agree without knowing everything that's involved in that consent form. Deciphering what these all mean is confusing for a person at any age, but as a teen, it's even harder to navigate the confusing legal texts that we've already agreed to.

Just about anyone with access to the internet can find out a lot of information about you with just a quick search online. Some of this information is what you've willingly put online, while the rest is information collected by data companies and marketing agencies who track your purchase (Teague, 2019). Social media apps like Instagram track how long you spend looking at posts (Keach, 2018). This information is collected and stored, and there's no telling how big your digital footprint will grow over time.

Whether they're using your phone number, full name, email address, or even just a sibling's information, those with the right motives can find out many bits and pieces of personal information about you. The reason that somebody might want this information is endless as well. They might be complete strangers from different parts of the world who want to steal your personal information for financial gain. They might want to open up new credit cards or take out loans in your name. They might try to steal your credit card balance, your bank account information, or other very valuable monetary aspects of your life that could have devastating results.

During youth, you can't know if certain things are going to come back to haunt you in the future. When you're applying for a job or a scholarship for college, you don't know if something you posted when you were 12 years old is going to come back and make you look bad.

Even if you use fake names, don't show your face in your profile picture, and don't reveal any personal information, as there are people out there who can gain access to your personal and private information if they really want to. As much as you might feel as though you know about internet privacy, there's always somebody else who knows more and who has worse intentions.

This information is not meant to scare you. We don't have to be afraid. We don't have to avoid social media altogether, forever. It's just important that we are aware of just how much it can impact our privacy.

More than our health is put at risk when we get online. Teenagers are susceptible and vulnerable to creating a lasting digital footprint. The footprint we leave behind will never go away. It might change shape over time, but there are many websites that copy and store our information. Some of these websites do so automatically. For example, on a social media site like Reddit, you can post something online and delete it. When you go to read it, you don't see that post anymore. However, there are multiple different sites that automatically copy all of this information and save it in an archive so that you can still view certain deleted posts.

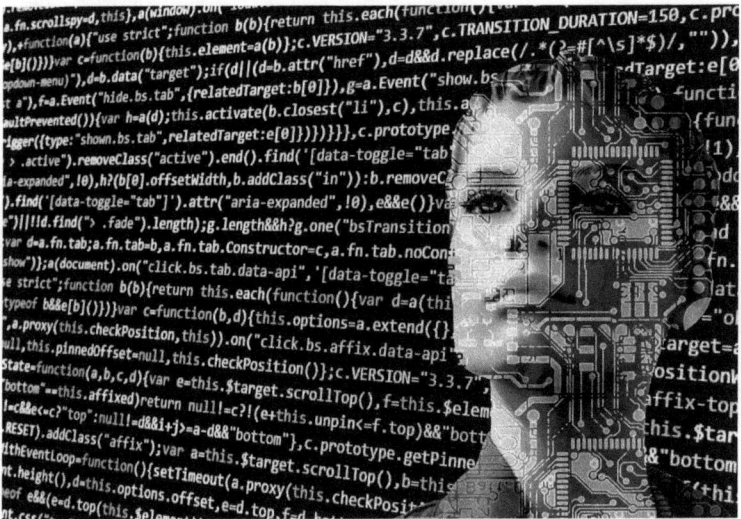

You never know if what you post is going to come back to haunt you, and you never know just how different your beliefs might be in the future. Old tweets have cost some people their jobs, scholarships, and more, so it's best to maintain a clean image online. Any celebrity or internet personality that you follow likely has some sort of scandal where past tweets or Instagram posts were uncovered, making them look bad. At the time, these posts weren't necessarily made with malicious intent, but people changed their beliefs over time. Many things that were once culturally and socially acceptable are now rightfully deemed offensive. While it certainly was offensive at the time, it was still deemed more acceptable, so people got away with that kind of behavior.

Nowadays, it's hard to tell what kind of casual language or belief systems we're using that is going to quickly become outdated and hurt our image down the line. You might post something seemingly acceptable, but later, as you age, you uncover more truths about how it really comes off.

Over time, our data is collected in every corner and stored away on the internet. It's best to make sure that what you're putting out there is something that you will always be proud of or at least unashamed of.

You likely won't regret posting pictures of your pets, and you likely aren't going to feel ashamed or embarrassed for sharing some of your thoughts or emotions. Even selfies are generally harmless. However, the frequency and amount can greatly impact your digital footprint.

Blue Light

Aside from the risks to your privacy, it's also important to raise awareness of the dangers of blue light. Blue light is a specific digital light that "can penetrate the eye's natural filters and cause damage to the retina ("Why Your Teen," n.d.)."

The artificial light that we are exposed to all day long can really mess with our circadian rhythm, which is the natural cycle that our body goes through. It's why we feel more alert during the day and more tired going to bed at night. Naturally, our circadian rhythm follows the sunlight. Humans are diurnal, which means that we sleep when it's night and we are awake when the sun is out. You've likely heard of nocturnal animals before. Well, humans are the opposite.

Sometimes we still sleep when the sun rises. Sometimes we go to bed even before the sun sets. But for the most part, humans are *not* nocturnal. Diurnal animals include ducks, bears, and whales. Nocturnal animals include owls, bats, and raccoons.

Despite our differences, we all follow a circadian rhythm that is triggered by light.

When the sun sets, that means some animals should head to bed while others start the hunt. When the sun rises, some animals scurry to their homes while others begin to awaken. Whether we are nocturnal or diurnal changes some of our biological functions. For example, some nocturnal animals have the vision to see at night which allows them to hunt better. Humans can't see in the dark because we're not supposed to be doing regular things in the dark.

Artificial light triggers these biological responses as well. When the light suddenly turns on, you might wake up. If somebody comes bursting into your room and turns the switch on, that's enough to wake you up in the morning. While you might not feel alert and refreshed, it's still a signal to you that now is the time to awaken. This is because even when our eyes are closed, our eyelids are thin enough to be able to sense the light that's around us. When it's really dark, you might feel more tired. If you're in a movie theater or cuddled up on the couch with your pet and blanket at night, you might feel a little bit more sleepy because it's dark and peaceful.

Artificial light messes with our circadian rhythm so when we are in our beds using our phones late at night after the sun has set, our bright phone can trick our brain into thinking it's daytime.

A flashy, colorful phone that is making noise is not telling your brain that it's time to go to bed. It's telling your brain that it's time to be awake and alert. Our phones also emit light even when we aren't using them through different notifications. Constant use of your phone is going to mess with your body's natural biological system and confuse those natural triggers.

This causes us stress, therefore having a greater impact on our health. Blue light can also cause eyestrain. Eyestrain alone can cause headaches but also the act of not getting enough sleep or having disrupted sleep can also increase your chance of having a headache.

As you are a teen, you're likely even more susceptible to these negative side effects since your body is still developing. Blue light also stops and reduces the production of melatonin (Summer, 2023). Melatonin is one hormone that gets released when it gets darker, especially when nighttime comes around. Melatonin helps to calm you down and make you feel more rested. When your melatonin and other hormones are messed up, then you're not going to feel tired enough to get a deep sleep.

Even if you are not using your phone and getting in bed at a decent time, excessive social media use close to bedtime can still impact your hormones, therefore impacting your sleep.

As a developing teen, getting rest is incredibly important so that you can function. If you find that you're struggling to pay attention, or you feel extremely tired throughout the day, there's a good chance that blue light has been impacting you. Our phones are not the only devices that emit blue light either. Watching TV, and using tablets, laptops, and desktop computers can all emit blue light. As you can see, it's not just the act of using social media that can have a negative impact, but also the act of using a phone or device at all.

The Impact on Mood

Aside from the basic risks and blue light effects that excessive social media and cell phone use can have in your life, these things can also greatly impact your mood. Social media use can trigger our body's natural stress response (Mastroianni, 2020).

Like the circadian rhythm, we all have a biological feature wired within us for survival. This is the stress response, also known as the fight-or-flight response. Whenever we are presented with a perceived threat, we have two common reactions: to flee the scene or to attack the threat.

The flight response is why birds and pigeons will simply fly away when you approach a group of them pecking around on the ground. The next response is to fight the threat. This is why animals like snakes or spiders might attack you when they feel cornered.

There are other types of responses to stress as well. One is the freeze response. You can think of this through the example of a deer or a possum freezing in the beam of your headlights when you're driving on the road at night.

There are other responses, like the fawn response, where the threatened person tries to please the threat. For example, a student who is bullied might try to impress their bully in an attempt to ease up the level of abuse endured.

In terms of using your cell phone, the main stress response that you will feel is going to be the fight, flight, or freeze response. For example, if you see something really infuriating online, you might start going on rants or leaving angry comments in response to help alleviate some of the stress that you feel. You might freeze by socially isolating. You might turn your phone off and then just lie in bed and not talk to anybody. You might flee by closing one app and immediately opening another one, trying to ignore any stressful feelings or emotions by immediately distracting yourself with new content.

Most living things have a stress response, which is a chemical reaction that happens in your body. When you feel stressed, your heart starts to beat. Often, sweat will start to produce at a more frequent rate. You might also notice that you have trouble breathing or regulating your heart rate. All this can lead to even more stress, therefore creating an endless cycle. The fluctuation of the content that we see online can also seriously impact our mood. At one point, you're watching something hilarious and laughing to yourself in bed, and the next moment you are crying because you just saw the saddest video of a poor little abandoned animal who no one will adopt. After that, you're enraged and infuri-ated because you learned about something in history that seems unfair and unjust, and then you see videos of food and artwork that you want to consume and purchase. This can all happen within a matter of *10 minutes* and that is a lot of emotions to experience all at once, especially as a developing teenager.

We also have to think about *how* we use social media and *when* we use it. If you wake up first thing in the morning and start your day off by looking at enraging content or things that make you upset, then this is going to impact your mood for the rest of the day. You might get consistently triggered throughout the day, therefore feeling stressed and tired through every hour. The stress of social media isn't some-thing that just stays stuck in your mind either. It can start to make the rest of your body feel sick. You might grind your teeth or notice that you have really tense shoulders and even a tense jaw from the stress. You might even realize that it is impacting your digestive system. You might have trouble eating or maybe you feel nauseous before and after eating. While it feels like you're just emotionally experiencing some of the things you see on social media, it is constantly sending off internal signals in your body that are telling your brain to activate certain hormones.

When you are repeatedly activating the stress hormones, this will lead to a buildup of cortisol, and this impacts your cardiovascular and digestive systems. As you can see, the excessive social media use that we participate in is not just impacting our minds, it is having devastating results on our bodies as well.

Materialism

Excessive social media use can make us more materialistic. Studies show that an increase in social media use also increases feelings of materialism (Staloch, 2023). There are many advertisements online, and these rely on feelings of exclusivity and urgency to get you to make purchases. However, those signs have to be subtle. If a post says, "Buy this item because we want your money," you're not going to buy that item. However, consider an influencer doing a cleaning video. In one, brief shot, they show a cleaning product. They flashed the label really subtly, but it was long enough for you to see what they were using. You're more likely to purchase that item because you see it being used in a seemingly more authentic way. The methods that marketing agencies are using are very hard to catch nowadays, making us feel constantly pressured to make a purchase without realizing we're being sold something.

Seeing your favorite artists, musicians, actors, and influencers all using similar products or following a specific look creates a standard you might feel pressured to follow. When you can't access these things because they are sold out or too expensive, it's ultimately you who is left feeling as though you are not good enough.

A high level of social media use can cause an intense fear of missing out ("Is Your Phone," 2022). When we see people online with things that we don't have, it's hard to not feel as though there is something bigger, better, and more exciting that we are missing out on.

Raising awareness of these signs and symptoms does not make them go away overnight, but it can help you reduce the severity that they have on your mental health. The internet opens new doors to both good opportunities and potential risks.

Label Social Media Symptoms

Aside from social media use, the rates of depression and anxiety are still high among teens, with 40% of high school students reporting these mental health issues before 2020 (Weir, 2023). The pressures on teens, whether it's from social media or society in general, have always been hard.

One in three teens struggle with feelings of nervousness, anxiety, fatigue, irritability, and anger (Smith, 2022). Can you recall the last time you felt the same way? It's hard enough to manage school work and your social life, and on top of that, you have to figure out what you want to do with your future. Are you going to enter the workforce? Join the army? Go to college? What are you going to do once you get there? These pressures are endless, and it's a lot for a developing mind to handle.

The first thing to do to start reducing the impact of the emotional, mental, and physical effects of social media use is to label your emotions. Labeling your emotions is the act of putting a name to the thoughts and feelings that you are struggling with. Each behavior starts with a reaction. That reaction is the result of a thought or emotion that we have. If we can retrace our behavior back to those thoughts and emotions, we have better management over feelings, therefore it's easier to control our actions.

It can be hard to recognize the difference between controlling your emotions and responding appropriately. For example, have you ever had a classmate act out in the middle of class? They might have thrown something across the room or even physically harmed another student. You might have heard them say that they couldn't help it, or that they were upset. Our emotions are extremely valid. It's totally okay to be upset. It's completely normal and expected to be enraged or angry, especially when somebody does something that triggers you.

However, it is not okay to respond with violence or physical aggression. There's a difference between feeling the emotions that we have and what we choose to do with those feelings. Labeling is the way that you can stop those intense and seemingly out-of-control feelings from turning into destructive behavior.

Whenever you notice yourself wanting to participate in potentially harmful behavior, label your emotions. Having feelings and understanding your emotions are two different things. You can feel angry. You can feel annoyed. You can feel upset. What are you going to do with those feelings, though?

First, pick a specific word. Are you frustrated? Are you annoyed? Are you perturbed? When you're feeling angry, are you enraged? Are you disappointed? Are you offended? When you're feeling stressed out, are you overwhelmed? Are you overstimulated? Are you panicked?

All of these different words that were just used can mean very different things, even though sometimes those feelings can intertwine with each other and feel very similar.

Labeling your emotions is a way of untangling all of these thoughts that connect them.

Once you are able to label that emotion, you then know how to respond appropriately. If you're angry and overstimulated, it's important to walk away from the situation. If you're feeling hurt or upset, it's important to talk to the person who might have triggered that feeling within you. This is the first step in increasing mindfulness over our stress levels.

Self-reflection is a powerful tool that enables you to raise awareness over how you are thinking, reacting, and behaving in general. It becomes more of a natural habit to reduce your feelings and respond appropriately when you make it a priority in how you react and respond.

Whenever you are overcoming any form of addiction, self-reflection is crucial to stay one step ahead of your most debilitating thoughts and intrusive impulses. If you're feeling stressed, sad, or overwhelmed, you might have the urge to start binge eating or snacking. You might have the urge to procrastinate and ignore your responsibilities. Social media is an outlet that we might turn to in order to alleviate emotions, but social media then causes even more panicked feelings, perpetuating a cycle of undesirable behavior.

Make self-reflection a continued practice, then start talking to others about your feelings. Talk to your parents or your best friends. Find somebody who you feel safe with and express how you feel. You are not alone in the struggle, no matter how much it might feel that way. We often feel isolated and alone because we are so afraid of talking about our emotions. Chances are, members of your family and many of your friends also feel trapped by the stress of social media. Talking it out can help you make better sense of your emotions while also gaining more insight into the things that you're struggling with the most.

After you start to gain a better sense of your emotions, it's then important to start to label triggers. What is triggering you to want to reach for your phone? For example, you might find that you're constantly procrastinating. The stress of schoolwork could be a big trigger for you that makes you want to escape into social media. Another trigger might simply be being bored at home. You might not have enough to keep you busy at home or activities and outlets that you can dive into. When you don't have a car or money to go out and do things, it can feel as though there's nothing to do other than sit online. This can be another trigger that makes you want to start checking in with the world around you.

Another trigger might be the stress and anxiety of seeing other people's lives. Seeing somebody else's accomplishments might start to trigger your thoughts of self-deprecation. You might feel as though you are not good enough or that you don't have the same things they do. Identifying these triggers will make it easier for you to take control of your mindset. Write down your emotions and your triggers. Keep a journal to help you keep track of your thoughts so that you have something to go back to. This will help you track your progress and see that you are making change, while also helping to increase awareness of the things that continually trigger you. You can also write them down on paper to make them more real. Sometimes it's hard to make sense of everything that's going on in our minds, but when we put it down on paper in front of us, it's easier to see it. Keeping track of your thoughts creates a road map of your mindset. This will help you explore what has been going on in your mind on a deeper level.

Reminders

- **Step #2**: Recognize the dangers social media has had on your life.

Social media has been such an ingrained part of our everyday life since we were young, developing children. It's hard to realize just how dangerous and damaging it can be when everyone we know and interact with is using it seemingly as much as we are.

Not all social media is bad, but, according to The Mayo Clinic, heightened use of social media (three or more hours a day) is associated with a higher rate of mental health issues ("Tween and Teen Health", n.d.). Knowing how it's been impacting you will ensure you stay one step ahead of the control that it can have.

3. Reduce Phone Usage

Once you finally understand just how damaging this habit has been, you can then start to reduce usage overall to prevent experiencing more symptoms and decrease the impact it's had on your life.

The Time We Give to the Internet

Teens spend an average of seven hours on "screen media" per day (Rogers, 2019). How are your hours allocated? Whether you're spending time online watching your friends' stories or reading threads on interesting information, chances are, much of the time you spend online is filler content that doesn't necessarily provide extensive value or elicit positive emotions.

Other People's Lives

Society is so much different now than what it used to be. Teens hundreds of years ago would have been lucky to have a couple of close friends. Nowadays, we can be a part of many different types of groups. You might have a friend group specifically from your school. You might have a wider friend group and connect with people outside of your school district. You might have a specific online group of friends who you play a certain video game with. You might have social media friends who you interact with only online, never having met them in person.

Aside from just the people that we know and connect to, we also have access to the lives of complete and total strangers. From celebrities to influencers, you can tap into the personal lives of many different types of notable figures. You can see what they're wearing. You can see what they eat. They give you glimpses into their daily life, including their morning and night routines. You might know what their favorite breakfast is, and maybe you could recite some of their favorite movies or TV shows. We know what they watch and what they do with their free time. We know the lives of their pets, and there are some people who we have watched grow over the years. You might have been following an influencer who had a child and you recall the time that they announced their pregnancy and now their child is attending school. We have access to so much information about complete strangers who we will likely never come in contact with. A lot of the time that we spend online is spent watching the lives of other people.

Alternatively, some people watch *our* lives. They spend their time on the internet, keeping up with the things that we share. Whether or not this is a good thing is completely up to you. It's nice to stay connected. It's nice to have insight into how other people live their lives. Our natural curiosities lead us to want to know what other people are up to. However, we can waste a lot of time doing this, which leads to missed opportunities outside of social media coupled with lower self-esteem.

You might follow 100 different influencers and know the details of many of their different likes and interests. When you are in a certain friend group, what other people do with their time will likely bleed into what you do with *your* time. You will likely have similar interests. You might have the same favorite band or maybe you go and see similar movies together. You might play certain games together and generally talk about the same things. That type of small social connection is expanded into the online world. Now, you might be influenced by the people who you follow. You watch what they like, you take their suggestions for food and clothing, and it can feel as though you're much closer to them than you actually are. This can create a parasocial relationship, where we feel as though they are a bigger part of our lives than they really are. Social media offers an intimate look into somebody's life. You see things that you wouldn't have been able to see years ago. Celebrities have always been a point of fascination, but nowadays we know a lot more about them. You used to have to wait for the next magazine to come out to figure out what certain celebrities were up to. The only way that we had access to what they were eating was through interviews and other types of videos. Whether you are lying in bed at night, or sitting bored in a classroom, you can open your phone and check social media to see what people are up to. This accessibility can make it hard to look away. It makes it a bigger part of our lives, so when these celebrities go through hard periods, controversies, and other stressful events, it might impact us much more than it should.

Following influencers and celebrities is not a bad thing. It's fun to have people you like and follow, and many provide us with entertainment. It's not a bad thing to have people that we like following, in general. It's also not a bad thing to be influenced. Sometimes you want to be able to trust somebody's opinion and know what types of recipes are good or where a good place to buy quality clothing might be. However, if we're not carefully navigating that relationship, it can become very influential in the way we think and the way we feel.

Advertisements

Children under three years old cannot tell the difference between ads and regular videos ("Advertising," n.d.). This means they are more likely to be influenced by subliminal messages and hidden manipulation tactics.

We are constantly bombarded with advertisements. In fact, it was estimated in 2006 that adolescents are exposed to over 40,000 advertisements every year (Strasburger, 2006). It's hard to tell just how much more that has increased over the last couple of decades.

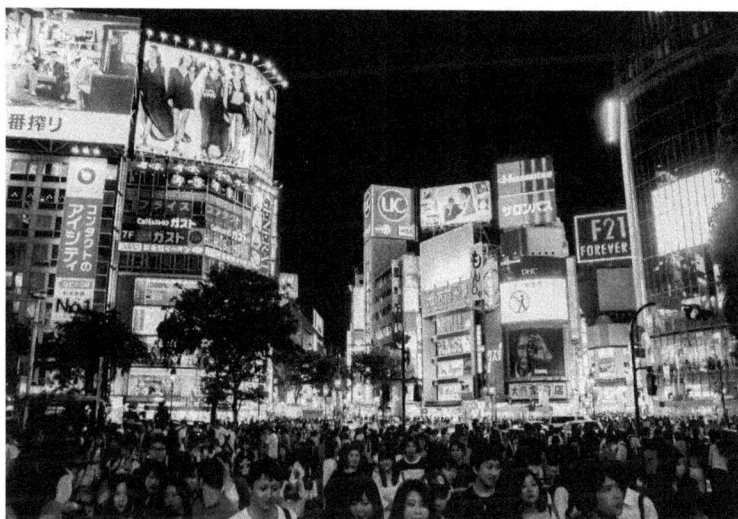

Advertisements are what keep the internet running. Without them, everything would be far less profitable. Social media would not be a billion-dollar industry if it weren't for advertisements.

However, advertisements all have a purpose. They all have an intention. They all exist to specifically influence you to spend your money. They want you to buy into a certain lifestyle or belief.

Advertisements aren't just based on one person's idea either. There are teams filled with psychological and marketing experts that exist specifically to make a product more appealing.

There are many different types of advertisements. First and foremost, we have obvious advertisements. These are things like forced ads. You might have to watch a 30-second clip before you can continue watching a video. Then, there are very subtle forms of advertisements. These are often disguised to look like more natural product placement. You will see this mostly through influencer advertising. For example, somebody might be using specific products in their video and talking about how great they are. You'll see this a lot in makeup tutorials or cleaning videos. Some of these are still very obvious as the tone of the video might shift and there will be links to buy the product. They also have to include disclaimers on different websites if something is being sold. However, not everybody pays attention to these small, subtle cues, so it can feel a lot more natural when you see somebody using a product in their day-to-day life.

Sometimes advertisements are even disguised as viral videos. There are brands and marketing teams behind them to make them look as though they're funny or extreme videos, but ultimately, you'll end up seeing an advertisement in the background through a poster on a wall or a T-shirt that somebody might be wearing.

Teens are especially targeted by advertisements because they have a lot of spending power. Many teens have access to their parents' finances, whether they have their own credit card or a shared bank account. Many teens are also working jobs and they don't have as many financial responsibilities like rent and utilities, therefore they have more disposable income. If you're working a part-time job after school, you might be putting some away in your savings, but you still have a lot of spending power when it comes to smaller prod-ucts like drinks and snacks. On top of this, teenagers have lower impulse control and media literacy. Somebody who is 45 years old might have 10 times as much money as you, but they are also a lot more aware of the manipulative and intrinsic behavior that advertisements have. As a teenager, you might not be as aware of just how tricky some of these marketing tactics are, and how obviously they're being used against you.

The best way to reduce how many ads you see is to use ad blockers. There are also paid versions of different apps that help block advertisements as well. When you do see an ad, it's crucial that you look at what the intention of it is before you let it influence you. What is being sold to you and who is profiting off of the sale? Advertisements are meant to make life look much better on screen than it is in real life, and therefore the real life around you seems bleak and boring. This makes you want to buy that product. It creates this false sense that maybe if you just purchase the thing that they are showing you, perhaps your life will look a little bit more like the advertisement you see on screen.

Advertisements also try to sell us promises. They use authority and trusting tactics so that you believe them. Aside from trying to sell specific products, advertisements also exist for brand awareness. Large companies want to make sure that their product is seen in subway stations, on billboards, in commercials, and through music streaming apps. Even though they might not be selling you a specific product, they're still creating brand awareness. Then, when you're in the store and you're looking at five different brands to choose from for a specific product, you are swayed to purchase the one whose advertising has been most prominent. You've seen that product a lot, therefore you feel as though it's more trustworthy, making you more inclined to make that purchase. It's essential that we stay ahead of the urges and temptations created through advertisements so that we don't fall for their manipulative tactics.

Upsetting News

Advertisements drive the internet. To see those advertisements, you still have to click on entertaining and intriguing content. This is done through sensationalized videos, viral headlines, and clickbait.

Sensationalized news is very clickable, and most websites know this. All it takes is a headline that reads something like, "Crazy Man Does Crazy Thing," and it gets you to want to click on it and find out what exactly it was that he did. Then, once you click on that page, you're bombarded with 50 different advertisements throughout that are typical on the right and left-hand side, as well as through pop-ups. Professionals are hired to create these sensationalized headlines, and copywriters are very skilled in making something that is a little more mediocre seem very intriguing.

In addition, not everybody is going to read the full article, so writers try to jam as much as they can in the headline, as well as in the first few sentences. What this means is that we are left consuming anxiety-inducing news all day long that has been presented in a very stressful way.

For example, you might see an article that's titled, "Scientists Discover New Life Form." They use a picture of an alien as the cover photo, and the heading underneath asks, "What does this mean for our future?" All of a sudden, your brain might start thinking about aliens or other odd creatures. In reality, once you read the article, it's a new variant of a different type of fungal microorganism that they already knew existed. In reality, they don't really know much about it, so while it's still a fascinating discovery, it's not the same thing as finding an actual alien on another planet. This is just one example of how a small news story can get inflated into a crazy conspiracy or theory.

When you see just the headlines and you're absorbing all these sensationalized things all day long, it can make the world seem very crazy and stressful. This adds to some of the panic and anxiety that you might be feeling when consuming other things. Doom scrolling refers to how we sometimes consume news and headlines in an excessive way. Even though we know it's making us feel bad and we know that it's never-ending, we might continue scrolling and reading very upsetting and triggering things.

There's always going to be interesting information out there. There's always going to be a story about somebody doing something crazy. There's always going to be stories about how the government is corrupt or science is scary. There's never going to be a shortage of stressful news because life is stressful. However, when that's all you're consuming all day long, it can make the world seem like a very scary or depressing place, and that will contribute to your mindset, even when you're not using your cell phone.

Repetitive Content

A lot of the content that we see online is also extremely repetitive. You've likely seen the same meme or funny video 10 times. After a while, it loses its humor, and you might have not even thought it was that entertaining in the first place. However, because of the way that we're able to share content, you might end up seeing the same thing over and over again.

We can also consume hundreds of images at a time or within a social media scrolling session, so you might forget that you saw it the first time around, then you see it again, and again and again, and it then becomes ingrained in your memory and loses all meaning. How many times have you had the same video sent to you by a friend? Since our algorithms are similar to our friends' and those of the people that we interact with online, chances are, they're getting served the same things that we are. When we are constantly viewing the same kind of content, it can make us feel like we are wasting time.

In real life, outside of the screen, we likely repeat the same content. You listen to the same songs that you like or you restart your favorite series once finished. However, when you see all these repeated things online, it's usually because it's simply what you're getting served and not necessarily based on the fact that you are willingly seeking this information out.

We can't always help what content we're fed, but this certainly eats away at the free time that could be better spent elsewhere.

How to Start Reducing Screentime

The average American checks their phone up to 352 times a day (Waltower, 2023). It's hard to know exactly how much everyone checks their phone, though, as screen time is tied up with work and education. We have to check emails and messages, especially if we are talking to bosses and coworkers. However, even without notifications, it's estimated that most people "check their phone every 15 minutes (D'Onfro,

2018)." Do you drink water this much? Do you get up and stretch your legs this much? There's nothing quite like phone usage, and while it is sometimes necessary to check in online, most of the time, our quick check-ins lead to distraction and wasted time.

Make It Less Enticing

One way to help reduce your screen time is to make phone usage less enticing. Phones are so addictive because, well, they are fun. They're like little video games in our hands (and often they do allow for gaming). They have colorful lights. They have fun buttons that make noises when you click on them. You can do anything that you want with a phone. They make you feel powerful.

They present you with endless opportunities, and when you get bored with one thing, you can close an app and open another. Because of this accessibility and fun usage, it's very hard to put our phones down. One way to make this less enticing is to turn your screen to black and white. Indeed, you can use grayscale, a feature that is often built into our actual phones. Grayscale will remove some of the bright colors and fun images that we see, making the phone screen's content visually less appealing.

Brains crave color. It's something that's been naturally wired into us as a survival tactic. Thousands of years ago when we didn't have access to the grocery store, we had to go out and hunt for our food. Foraging meant finding berries and seeds, as well as mushrooms and other types of fungi in the wild. All of these things are a little bit more colorful. When you're walking by a bush, you're going to notice when it has berries on it. When you're walking by a tree, you're going to notice when it has mushrooms growing off of it. When you are walking through a grassy plane, you're going to notice the flowers. These things are food sources, so we have been wired to be able to visually see color and then feel pleasure and happiness once we see this color.

When you're scrolling on your phone all day long, you're very overstimulated by all of this constant design. There are many psychological theories about color as well, and app developers know this. For example, blue is calming and supposed to be very friendly. Think about how many blue apps you might have on your phone. Colors like yellow or orange might be seen as a little bit more cheerful. Purple can be more creative. Color is used against you to elicit certain types of emotion. To block that type of manipulation, you can then turn the color off on your phone. You can still scroll through social media. You can read interesting articles, and you can watch funny videos. Once the color is removed, it makes it a little bit less stimulating and enticing for your brain, therefore helping you to slowly reduce usage over time.

Another way to make phones less enticing is to delete all of your apps except for the ones that are needed for work or school. In our modern society, many companies want you to download apps so they can track your purchases and send you notifications. They want you to have their restaurant information so you can easily place food orders. Shopping apps want you to download them so that they can track your online activity, therefore making it easier to provide you with targeted ads. The thing about these apps, however, is that they also send notifications. When you're sitting there bored at school and you get an app saying that there's a 25% off sale at your favorite store, or that there's a buy-one-get-one-free deal from your favorite restaurant, that automatically triggers you to want to consume. Deleting these apps will reduce your notifications and make them less enticing altogether.

You can still place online orders through your phone's web browser, and you can still shop online when you want. However, removing apps removes an important force of influence.

Another way to make social media use less enticing is to unfollow certain people on the internet who do not make you happy, bring you joy, or make you feel good. If anyone triggers you or causes stress, it's best to click the "unfollow" button and move on. Whether you are on TikTok, Instagram, or another social media app, it's crucial to go through who you're following to see if they're actually making you feel good about yourself and if you want to continue keeping up with them.

Unfortunately, it can be hard to let go of certain people, especially if you've been watching them for a long time, but you have to really evaluate if they are people who are making you feel good and providing value to your life. You can even unfollow people who you know in your personal life. You don't have to stay connected to somebody just because you've already established an online relationship with them. If you went to school with somebody five years ago, but you've never seen them since, it's okay to let them go. Just because they're following you doesn't mean that you have to follow them back. If you're not ready to unfollow somebody, it's also perfectly acceptable to simply block their activity so that they don't pop up in your news feed.

Another tactic to make your phone less enticing is to make it physically restricted. One way to do this is to use painter's tape. Put a piece of painter's tape across your phone screen. Put your phone in a plastic sandwich bag. Wrap some string around your phone and tie it in hard knots. When you want to reach for your phone, that small physical thing is a little reminder that you don't need to be using it right now. Our phone usage can be so automatic that we reach for it without even thinking. When you go to grab your phone and realize that there's a little piece of painter's tape over the screen, that's a reminder that tells you *Oh yeah, I'm trying to reduce this activity.* When you have a plastic bag over your phone, you can still see necessary notifications pop up if needed, so if your mom texts you to let you know she'll be late coming home from work, you can still see that text and not feel panicked when she doesn't show up on time. However, if you get a bunch of notifications about things that don't matter, it's a lot harder to navigate your phone when it's inside the plastic, therefore, you're less likely to use it.

Make It Less Accessible

On days when you really can't help but look at your phone, make it less accessible. In addition to making it less exciting, it's time to make it hard to even reach. Put it up high on a shelf that requires a stepladder, then put the stepladder away. You're less likely to want to go and reach for your phone when you have to go through the process of getting the stepladder back out. When you make a multi-step process to get the phone, then you are more likely to not want to use it. Another great way to make it less accessible is to put the passcode in incorrectly several times so that you become locked out. When you're locked out of your phone, you can still make emergency phone calls, so if something really bad happens and you do need to call for help, you will have access to that. However, you can lock your phone for 15 minutes or an hour or more, so that if you have to study or do some household chores, you will not have access to it.

This is also a great way to get you to do things like read or exercise more. You can lock your phone for 30 minutes or an hour, spend that time working hard, and then when that time is up, you have access to your phone again, and it becomes a little reward.

Consider other methods to keep you from your phone like putting it in another room or getting a timed lockbox to keep it in. You can put it in a kitchen cabinet downstairs while you work upstairs, making it harder to get to. You could also try giving it to a sibling or a parent to hide and let them know that you are trying not to use it until a specific time. Then, once that time comes, they can let you know where they hid it.

You can also consider letting the battery die so that when you're trying to study, your phone is dead, and you can't even turn it on and pick it up. This means that you won't have access to any phone calls or be able to make an emergency call, so only do this when somebody else is around just to make sure that you have an emergency contact if needed. Lastly, consider using a long and complicated passcode rather than face recognition. Make it complicated and change it weekly. Write it down and hide that piece of paper so that it's more challenging to try to get into the phone.

The less accessible and exciting your phone is, the less likely you are to spend too much time on it.

Reminders

- **Step #3**: Reduce how much time you spend on your phone.

You don't have to give up on your phone altogether. You don't have to demonize phone usage or feel guilty about the desire to stay tuned in online. The important thing to remember is to start to utilize methods of making your phone less enticing and accessible so you can put more focus on the things that really matter. One good way to help you kick-start this new period of social media reduction is to first do a temporary cleanse.

4. Take a Break

Sometimes just reducing phone use isn't enough, and while it's good to cut back on how much time you spend online overall, the next crucial step is to take a complete break from social media altogether.

Social media connects us to other people, and that's arguably a good thing. However, when we are not in the right mental head space, we might start to follow certain pages and look at specific posts a bit longer than others, and those become a part of our online profiles, impacting our algorithm. The Center for Brain Health puts it perfectly by saying:

- *"The impact of social media is minor for most people; the platform recommends friending people you might know and tailors the tone and content of posts and advertisements to suit your preferences. However, social media platforms need to be more discerning about the types of interests they use to connect with people. This can lead to severe problems when people interested in armed revolution or communal violence are automatically shown content that solidifies their beliefs and connects them with like-minded people nearby* (Chapman et al., 2021)"

Essentially, if you feel depressed and anxious, you'll get fed content that perpetuates this mindset, making those emotions worse. Each time you log on, your negative beliefs or bad mood becomes more solidified, making it harder to see anything else but the perceived truth presented on your phone. This can impact us in many different ways:

- If you like shopping and spend too much money on clothes, you're fed even more advertisements and "deals," making you feel as though you should be spending your money on these things.
- If you fall under the belief that you hate other people and the world is filled with criminals, villains, and other evil beings, you'll get fed stressful news about people committing heinous acts.
- If you believe we should all just work hard to get rich and that life is all about making money, having luxury cars, and living in mansions, you will get fed this type of content, solidifying this belief system.

When we are presented with information that challenges these beliefs, it can make us feel anxious and overwhelmed. Social media creates our belief system and then upholds it by feeding us specified algorithms. When we are unaware of this, it can have grave effects on our minds and bodies.

Your Mind Off Social Media

Research proves that when we limit social media use, it can result in (Malouff, 2023):

- lower levels of depression
- less loneliness
- improved relationships
- better psychological effects

Because everyone uses social media in their own way, we all feel these impacts in individualized ways as well. Knowing some of the benefits of staying off social media can help you recognize just how important it is to reduce screen time.

Reduced Stress

Whether you are dealing with your own conflict or just sitting in the front seat of someone else's drama, there is a lot of stress that can come from spending too much time online.

Excessive phone use can create a sense of urgency. When you receive notifications, they use sounds like dings and bells, and that makes you feel more alert. It makes you feel as though there's some sort of urgency that you need to pick up your phone and check in on. Everything that we see online can elicit different types of emotions. If you see somebody posting about an amazing new purchase they have, that can make you feel jealous. If you see somebody posting about their amazing partner or a group of friends, it can make you feel lonely. All of these emotions that we experience throughout the day can add up and really impact our level of stress. This excessive stress can make us very sensitive. It makes us more focused online and less focused on the world around us. Then, when you feel all of the natural life pressures adding up, it makes them even harder to deal with. For example, let's say you find that you've been spending four hours on social media, you finally put your phone down and decide to get to work on your homework.

However, as you're sitting there, you start to feel a higher sense of urgency, and you start to feel overwhelmed by impending deadlines. All of the good feelings you had scrolling social media have gone away, and now the rush of the stress of schoolwork suddenly floods your mindset. You're looking at your schoolwork and you've realized you haven't studied enough. You haven't completed as much as you thought you would. It makes life feel even more stressful when you're already focused elsewhere and giving less attention to the things that actually require your attention. This can also make us more sensitive to feedback. When we're feeling insecure and like we're not good enough, it makes us feel like we're inadequate. This will make it harder to take criticism. When you get a bad grade in school, it might make you feel even worse because of the excess stress that's already been built in your body through high levels of social media use. This also contributes to us being more easily triggered by stress.

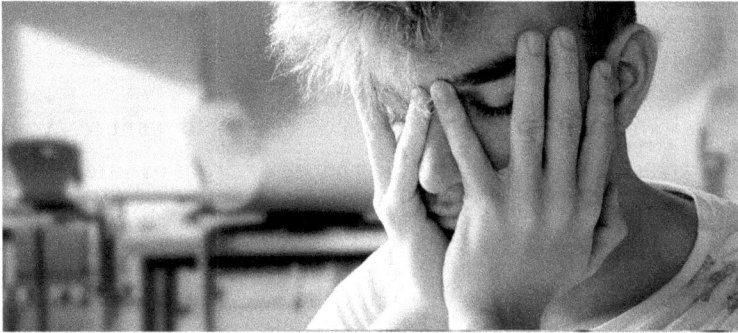

Stress is triggering for anybody. It's very fair to feel over-whelmed by any of life's demands. However, when you are experiencing high levels of cortisol and other stress hormones in your body when real-life stressors do arise, it can make them feel 10 times worse. We can also feel stressed from excessive social media use because we feel bored or empty without the use of our phones. It can be harder to focus in the real world and stay present on the things that require our attention when we feel as though the internet is more interesting, and like we are missing out on things happening online.

This leads to a lack of focus, therefore, you might start to struggle with your schoolwork, and you might find that it's difficult to pay attention in class during lectures. Because of this lack of focus, you don't retain the information as well or comprehend the lessons when you're actually trying to do your homework or research papers.

You might find that it's really hard to focus on assignments and studying when you are outside of the classroom. Then what happens is your grades start to fail, and all of this homework becomes even more difficult to complete, therefore, you feel even more stressed out because of your lack of focus or excessive demands from school.

This can lead to procrastination. It's easier to want to avoid the stressors and do something more exciting or interesting rather than deal with all of the difficult things in life. All of this stress impacts our developing minds. Stress can also be triggered by the types of things that we see online. Even if you're not actively participating in fights or conflicts on the internet, you are still witnessing that stress from other people. For example, you might see a controversial video, and then in the comment section, there are many other people discussing this conflict. They might even make reaction videos and response videos and before you know it you are in a rabbit hole of some corner of the internet, learning about the intricacies of this drama. Though you might not be an active participant, you're still likely having arguments in your mind or going through conflict internally. You might be just witnessing the aggression from other people and that can bleed into your life and increase stress levels.

When you start to feel stressed out or even aggressive online, that will carry with you to the real world. You might find yourself having short tempers and more conflict with the people around you. Going through a detox from social media will help you reduce stress. It will help you clear your mind and become more focused on the things that matter.

More Free Time

There's often this feeling that we never have enough time. What you might come to discover is that once you are offline, you have plenty of extra hours in the day that you can dedicate to the things you love and have more passion for. Excessive social media use can result in decreased cognitive abilities, attention, and focus (Fotuhi, 2020).

It takes a lot of time to scroll through all of our social media platforms and profiles. By the time you're done checking one, another one has loads of new content, allowing you to endlessly scroll and be entertained through just the use of your phone. When you cut down on phone use, you'll then free up a lot more personal time, therefore, you have time to give to hobbies and things that actually interest you. This will lead to excessive amounts of productivity. Whether you are trying to get in shape, improve a physical skill, or want to study more and learn, you will find that you have more time to give to your passions and interests when you unplug.

On the one hand, you simply have more time because you are spending less time on the Internet. 30 minutes of social media time can become 30 minutes of reading. On the other hand, you will also save time because you will be more focused, therefore boosting productivity.

When you are less stressed out and you are thinking more clearly, it's easier to be productive when you're actually sitting down and reading. Trying to read in the middle of using your cell phone could mean only getting through a certain number of pages within 30 minutes. However, when you detox from social media and completely shut off from the internet, you might find that you're reading twice the speed. When you are more productive, you save even more time. There's also less urgency, meaning you can actually take things slowly and at the right pace. For example, if you're spending two hours on social media at night and then you have to study for an hour afterward, you might feel this great sense of urgency. You are trying to rush through all of your homework and get studying done as fast as you can. Then tomorrow when the test comes around, you realize that you didn't actually retain any of that information because you were speeding through the book. However, if you're able to actually sit down for those three hours and study, you find that you get your work done earlier, and you retain that information effectively because you don't have the panic and stress looming behind you. You'll also have more creative thinking skills and the ability to think more logically. This is because you will become less dependent on your phone. When you're sitting there and trying to figure out a problem, you might reach for your phone and Google the answer. You don't even have to think about the solution because your phone just has it for you. However, if you are less dependent on your phone, then you force yourself to use your thinking skills and try to come up with a solution on your own. If you are an artist and you're trying to think of something creative, you might use AI or other forms of inspiration online to help you think of ideas. When you are forced to think creatively, your perspective is going to be a little bit more unique.

Increased Health

Social media can reduce cravings and urges to binge and increase our sleep quality. Extra time spent reducing stress, taking care of hygiene, and even exercising are all additional benefits we might experience once we take the plunge and unplug.

All of these benefits that happen mentally are going to physically impact us in a positive way as well. When you are more focused and more productive, that decreases your stress level. When you're actually getting your homework done and participating in hobbies that you enjoy, you will be happier. You'll be more focused, therefore, you're going to start getting better grades and realize that you're more successful in your endeavors. You'll have more time to exercise. You'll have more time to hang out outside. You'll have more time to spend with friends and create stronger and more meaningful connections. All of this will lead to alleviated feelings and more inner peace and clarity. This will impact your health. You'll notice that it's easier to take care of yourself when you feel good about yourself and you're taking good care of yourself. This increases your body image and you'll also start to see yourself in a more positive light.

As a teenager, your body is still developing. You're growing. You're changing shapes. You're changing appearances. If you're not taking care of yourself in the right way, then as an adult you might find that you struggle with your health. You might struggle with maintaining a healthy body weight. You might find that you suffer from headaches, joint pain, and body aches because you're not getting enough physical movement. You might find yourself feeling depressed and lonely because you're not spending enough time outside or socializing with your friends.

There are many different layers to our health and social media absorbs so much of our time we start to neglect our physical anatomy. By reducing the time that you spend online, you will start to have more attention and care that you can give to taking care of your body and maintaining your physical health.

The 7-Day Detox and 30-Day Challenge

The first challenge to do is to take a 7-day detox. Sometimes it's hard to take the plunge because we feel as though we have to give up a big part of our life. One way to help this mindset is to shift your way of thinking to see it as a chance to regain lost time (Green, 2023).

If you can't do a 7-day detox, then it might be a sign that something more serious is going on. It's okay to reach out and ask for professional help if you believe it is needed! There is more at stake than just wasted time if you don't learn to reduce social media use. Your health is at risk when too much time is spent online.

Steps to a 7-Day Detox

Social media elevates our dopamine levels. For this reason, we might struggle with negative side effects as our bodies adjust to the lack of dopamine (Schubert, 2021). While that can be scary in itself, it's proof of just how important it is that we begin to reduce our social media dependency. Now is a time to find new sources of dopamine that will become long-lasting parts of your daily routine.

The first step to a 7-day detox is to identify your emergency source of contact. Many homes don't have landline phones anymore, so if there was some sort of emergency, you would need to be able to have a point of contact. Whether you need to call 911 or just check in with your parent, you will need to find some sort of emergency source that you can use to make contact during those seven days. If you have a parent who is frequently home, or even a sibling, then this can be the emergency contact. You can also enable voice-activated services on your phone, so if you are really in danger, you can put your phone somewhere nearby so that you can still call for help by voice prompts. You will likely not need to use your emergency contact, however, having one will provide peace of mind and reassurance that you do not need to check your phone.

The next part of the detox is to make your phone inaccessible by using one of the methods that was mentioned before. A great way to do this is through a timed lockbox.

Whatever you choose to use, the focus should be on simply making your phone inaccessible so that you can't reach for automatically.

Another great way to make it inaccessible is to simply make it unusable. If you make it unusable, then it's even easier to avoid reaching for it and automatically using it without you even realizing that's what you're doing. If you find that you are getting a new cell phone or device soon, and trading your old phone in, now might be the time to do that. You can simply deactivate your phone, delete all the apps, and then wait to reactivate the new one until you're done with the detox.

You can also consider trading your phone in for one that doesn't have as many smartphone features or purchase something like a flip phone so that you only have access to emergency services.

Another great way to make your phone less accessible and less enticing is to delete all your apps. Backup all of your information like any notes or photos, and then do a factory reset on your phone. You'll then be signed out of all of your devices so that you can't easily log into different apps. You can also consider changing your password to something that you don't remember. Do this for your email as well, write it down, and give it to a parent or a trusted friend for a temporary time so when you are ready to come back to your phone after that detox, they give you the password, therefore you can log into all of your apps once again.

You don't have to delete your social media accounts to do a detox. You can simply delete the app. You don't even have to deactivate the account. You simply have to remove the app from your phone so that you don't have the ability to open it. Then once you have figured out your plan for how you make your phone inaccessible, it's time to do the actual detox.

Make sure that it is a full seven days. This means Sunday night, put your phone away, and don't reach for it again until the following Sunday. The only time that it should be used is for emergencies only. If you are dependent on rides from your family members, talk about this plan with them and set up a very strict timeline so that they can pick you up after school and bring you home. Unless you have a job where you need your cell phone, then there really isn't another reason why you might have to check in online. You can use tablets or laptops to do schoolwork if necessary, and then after that, give your source of the internet away to a household member.

One important thing about doing the detox is to ensure that you have a plan in place for how you're going to replace the urge to check your phone. We become very dependent on our cell phones, so it can be hard to suddenly remove them. You might experience feelings of panic or stress. Your body is used to the use of your cell phone. You're used to those levels of dopamine and you're used to the habit of picking up your phone and holding it. If you lay in bed every night and watch TikTok, you're used to grabbing your phone and holding it with you before you fall asleep. You might find that it is hard to fall asleep at night because you don't have that routine in place anymore. When this difficulty arises, it increases the urge to break the detox. Resist impulses and know that this feeling will eventually pass.

Have something in place of that urge. When you remove something from your life that makes you feel good, your body is going to seek that out again. Your body wants to feel good, so suddenly now that source of good feelings is gone, you might start to panic and seek out other forms of instantly gratifying sources and substances. Having something in place means knowing exactly what to reach for when your social media impulses start to grow.

For example, this might be something like an exercise routine. You can download exercise videos to your desktop or laptop so that you can easily open them without having to navigate the Internet. You can go to the library and rent movies or books so that you have sources of entertainment that don't depend on the Internet. Have a craft or project that you want to work on. Buy some crochet books and crochet needles and try new patterns. Buy some paints and some blank canvases and explore your creativity. Get a notebook and a pen and paper and write down how you're feeling when you have the urge to reach for your phone. Start going on walks. When you want to just reach for your phone, instead, open your front door and go for a walk. It's still important to ensure that you let somebody know where you are going, and what time you expect to be home.

Invest in a record player so you can still listen to music without needing one of your electronic devices. Buy audiobooks on tape, or better yet, go to a live show where you can see performers share their art in person.

If you remove your phone from your life cold turkey, you find that you're going to struggle with impulsivity even more, so having a backup plan in place is always important to keep you focused through your downtime.

Steps to a 30-Day Free Challenge

Once you've completed your seven-day detox, you can participate in another challenge. This is the 30-day free challenge. All of the same rules apply. Make your phone inaccessible, have a point of emergency contact, and find somebody that you can depend on if you need rides or other forms of help throughout the process.

Going without social media for 30 days can be a lot harder, so in this case, you will likely want to deactivate your social media for the time being and make sure that everything has been deleted to reduce the urge to check-in. You can factory reset your phone and still use it for sending simple texts or making phone calls, but remember to try and make those only as needed. 30-day challenges are much easier if we have accountability partners.

Accountability partners are safe people with whom you can talk about this challenge, and they can help ensure that you stay on track with your goals. The best person to do this with is somebody who also wants to detox from social media. You and a sibling could even potentially share a phone for the time being so that you still can contact your parents or other relatives if needed, but you can hold each other accountable to make sure that nobody's checking in online or on their social media.

If you can challenge not just yourself but also another person who takes a break, it will be easier to stay true to this 30-Day Challenge. Having an accountability partner will also help reduce your fear of missing out. You can rest assured that you are not the only one who isn't tuning in online.

Another way to hold yourself accountable is to share it with the world. You might make a quick announcement saying, "Hey everybody, I'm going to be gone for 30 days. If you need me, contact [insert accountability partner]." You've likely seen it said before on social media posts about how someone is deleting their social media. While it might have induced an eye roll at the time, it can actually help you stay more accountable so that you're less likely to log right back on after taking a break. The more that you can stay consistent with this detox, the more likely you will see positive and beneficial results.

Reminders

- **Step #4:** Take some time away from social media.

Everyone can participate in a 7-day detox. You can set a 15-minute time period a day to check in with anyone you have to, like a parent that you might not live with. Other than that, you should challenge yourself to go a full week without social media use so you can discover the benefits on your own. Once you log back in, you'll find that you didn't really miss much of anything. Making social media breaks a regular part of your life can help you increase self-love.

5. Learn Self-Love

S ocial media can make us hate ourselves, so learning how to form healthy steps to self-care will increase self-love.

In life, when our phones come first, it's easy to let the negative thoughts and emotions that come with excessive screen time take the driver's seat in your mind. When this happens, it becomes even easier to neglect your health. Stress from social media combined with poor self-care results in even further negative side effects.

Understanding the importance of self-care begins with the acknowledgment and realization of all the ways it can impact your self-image.

Social Media and Self-Image

Social media can be very destructive to anyone's self-image, especially teenagers since they are still learning how to view the world and themselves.

Self-image is how we view ourselves. It's the opinions and beliefs we hold around our worth, whether that's through our intelligence, body, appearance, or skills. When you are constantly scrolling through social media, your mind is infiltrated with perfectly curated images presented by people who are only showing you what they want you to see. On top of that, there are many positive comments hyping up these unreal and edited images. Then, on the opposite end, you might see excessive hate and bullying. If someone looks remotely similar to you or is getting bullied for a similarity you both share, those words can hurt you just as much as the person whom the hatred is directed toward.

The constant comparison, reminders of what we don't have, and edited images can leave us feeling isolated and unskilled. As such, these are all things that can damage our mental and physical health.

Comparison

Social media has been proven to lower self-esteem, especially in teens 14 and younger (Bergman, 2023). Over 30% of teens felt shame toward their bodies, with some even stopping eating because of their level of worry ("Millions of Teenagers," n.d.).

Social media is incredibly damaging to a teen's developing mind because it provides an endless opportunity to compare themselves with others. Often, what ends up happening is that we make unfair comparisons, positioning our worst qualities against somebody else's best qualities. Comparison is hard because what it does is create a standard for how we think we should exist. When you are online and you see that somebody is living a certain lifestyle, it can make yours seem not as glamorous.

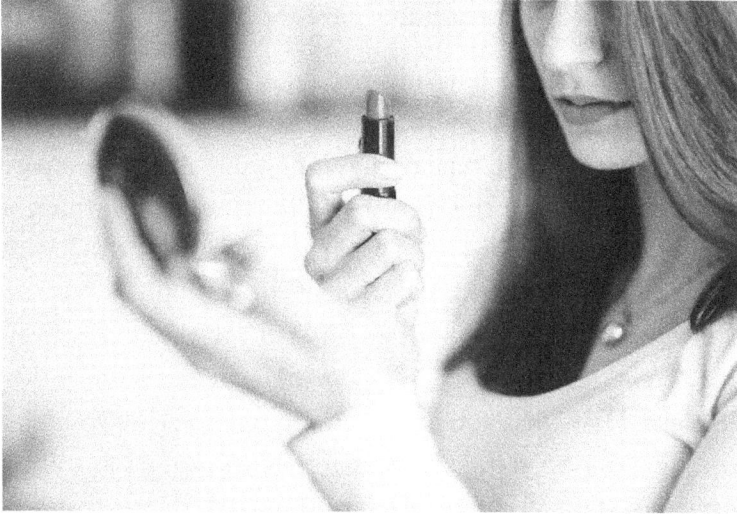

The thing is, when somebody takes a picture of their beautifully decorated apartment, they're not showing you the dirty garage. They're not showing you the other side of that room, where there is an unfinished paint job or stained furniture. They're only showing you the exact things that they want you to see.

Most humans are focused on their negative qualities in life. We are wired to pay attention to the small things that only we can see. Because of this, when you're scrolling online, you create this juxtaposition of *your* bad versus *their* good. A juxtaposition is the way that two things are positioned next to each other. When your worst qualities are positioned next to somebody else's best qualities, that can make you feel incredibly inadequate.

There's no one else to blame for our shortcomings but ourselves, so we end up hating ourselves and being resentful of our own appearances or lifestyles because we don't have the things that we feel as though we should have.

Comparison is also how advertisements are able to prey on our insecurities. When you see a perfectly filtered person holding up a certain type of makeup, suddenly you compare your own flaws to this very beautiful person. You think if you purchase that cover-up, you're going to be able to have a beautiful appearance just like them. In addition, we're also able to easily fixate on our flaws. When you take a selfie, you can zoom in on every little wrinkle, blemish, or other perceived flaw that you have. You can open a selfie you took on your phone and stare at it for hours, zooming in and cropping the picture, only focusing on the things that you don't like about yourself. When somebody else is scrolling through social media and they see your selfie, they likely just look at it for a few seconds and then scroll away. They're not sitting there zooming in to see that little crease you have next to your eyelid or that acne scar on your chin.

Do you do that to other people? Do you scrutinize somebody else's appearance in the same way that you do your own?

Chances are you likely don't. If you do, it's a sign that your body image issues have become so intense that they've shaped the way you perceive others as well. This comparison never helps us. It always leaves us feeling inadequate.

Comparison in general isn't always a bad thing. After you take a test at school, and you see that most of the class got an A while you barely passed, you might compare yourself. You think to yourself, *what did they do that I didn't?* This can help encourage you to study more next time. However, social media takes comparison to a whole new level, where we consistently focus on our shortcomings, leaving us feeling like we are never good enough.

What We Don't Have

Social media causes us to feel inadequate because of the things that we don't have. Since social media thrives off sales, we are bombarded with ads for things that we feel pressured to purchase, all while they are convincing us that we need them. When you see an ad over and over again telling you that you need a specific type of shoe or even a specific type of water bottle, of course, you're ultimately going to feel like you are not good enough because you don't have this thing that everybody else has. This includes products, clothes, and other things that make us believe they will give us the body image or lifestyle that we desire.

Humans are naturally wired to focus on inadequacies, flaws, and things that they don't have. This taps into our basic survival skills. When you're walking through the woods, you want to notice the spiders or snakes that are crawling around so that you stay protected. You're not as likely to pay attention to the beautiful sky or the intricacies of the leaves on a unique-looking tree. You're focused on negative aspects as a way to survive. We also fixate on blemishes for survival. If you notice that you have a rash or a bruise, you want to investigate what caused that to make sure that your health is protected.

However, that fixation on our flaws is taken to the extreme because of social media. When you are constantly focusing on the things that you don't have, you lose sight of all the amazing things that you actually do have.

One method to reduce this fixation is gratitude. Gratitude is a great way for us to appreciate the things that we actually have. Do you have a bed to sleep in every night? Do you have a bathroom where you can take a hot shower? Do you have a fridge with food that you can eat at any time you want? Do you have two legs to walk with or do you have two eyes to see with? Do you have two lungs to breathe with? Do you have a heart pumping blood? Do you have a brain that allows you to think logically? All of these things are things that we can be grateful for.

You can still have the desire to purchase certain things or live a certain lifestyle. However, when that desire becomes your focal point, you will always feel dissatisfied. You can still want to have certain clothes or other products: that's natural, and that's expected. You are human, after all, and you want to feel like you fit in and like you're a part of a group. However, when that is all you fixate on, it will leave you continually feeling inadequate and like your life is not worthy. Gratitude is a way to keep you balanced so that you can still emphasize the things that you are appreciative of. Do you have a family? Do you have parents who support you? Do you have siblings who you can hang out with? Do you have friends who make you laugh? All these things create an amazing life. We have to remember that some people don't have the things that we are grateful for, and those things we are grateful for can also get taken away at any time for reasons outside of our control.

You can log in to social media and see somebody post their beautiful house and luxury cars. But maybe they don't have anybody that they can feel safe around. Maybe they don't have anybody who loves them the way that your family and friends love you. Maybe there's something else going on in their life that we will never know about, so making a comparison to their life is very unfair to you and to all of the things that you have to be grateful for.

False Ideas

Now more than ever before, it is so easy to make fake content and put it online. Social media has built-in features so that you can smooth your skin and filter out any flaws. You can easily crop images so that you can make your life look more beautiful and appealing than it really is. This is harmful in two ways, though. The first way is because we are fed false information online. We are presented with fake images. We see beautiful people and we think we want to look like them, but even those people don't actually look like the images they're presenting online. They look much, much different.

In another way, it allows us to create our own false sense of reality. You can edit your body and your face to look much different than it actually does. You see that picture online and it makes you feel good because you believe that you are beautiful, as, now, you look like everyone else. Then, when you look in the mirror, or somebody else takes a picture of you and they don't edit it, it makes you feel even worse.

You start viewing the natural way that you actually look and thus you start feeling very inadequate. Anyone can take a selfie and put it through multiple different filters, high-lighting their best features and erasing the rest. Ultimately, this leaves the photo editor and everyone else who sees it feeling as though they are inadequate. It also makes us lose our sense of reality. As mentioned in the last section, you don't know what is truly going on in somebody's life. You don't know what they truly even look like. Most celebrities don't even look like the images that they post. They have professional teams who use very expensive software to make their skin look smooth and their facial features look more appealing.

Aside from photo editing, you can also use different angles. You can use perfect lighting to make your teeth look whiter than they are. You can make your body look different based on the position that you're in. Not everybody discloses all of the little tricks that they're using to make themselves look different, and social media is getting tricky when it comes to telling the difference between what is real and what is fake. You can even edit both prerecorded videos and live videos, so it's very hard to tell whether or not somebody actually looks like the images that they are portraying online. When you are comparing yourself and your life to a life that doesn't even exist, you will never feel satisfied. This increases your stress and makes it harder to appreciate yourself and love yourself for who you are.

Isolation

Because of the constant feelings of inadequacy and our shortcomings, it can be very easy to isolate ourselves from other people. Social media can make us feel very lonely.

When you are alone in your room under the covers and in the dark, it can be very lonely when you see somebody's social event. They might post a picture of themselves in a party setting where there are many people around them. You might see pictures of a group of friends all tagging each other, living experiences that you question if you'll ever have. This makes us feel very isolated, contributing to a negative self-image. When you isolate from other people, you start to get stuck in your own head. When you're stuck in your own head and constantly repeating negative things to yourself, you will ultimately be left feeling like you are not good enough. When you isolate, you start to lose out on opportunities. You might become distant in your friendships and check out of reality. However, just like we discussed in the previous sections, many people are portraying a false image online. For example, one trick that some influencers use is taking many different kinds of pictures on vacations or at a singular event. Then, rather than posting them all at once, they'll post them throughout the next month or two to make it look like they are doing something fun every weekend when, in reality, they took all of their pictures just within a couple of days.

You also have to consider that some people aren't actually enjoying these events. They are simply taking part in them because they want to have content to post online. It's important for us to stay checked in with reality so that we resist the urge to isolate and withdraw from others. It's okay to be alone. It's okay to not do everything that you see your friends doing. You are very young. You have a lot of life left to live. You will have plenty of experiences in the future. Just because it feels like your life is boring now or that you're not doing enough does not mean that this will be the case forever. Stay grounded in reality and focus on real life rather than the fake images that you see on the internet.

Successful Steps to Self-Care

It's so important today for teens to learn how to take care of themselves. Excessive social media use can negatively impact body image, and research shows that those who struggle with body image can be at a higher risk for suicide (Morin, 2022). The best way to combat poor self-image is through practical methods of self-care.

Our parents have to provide us with plenty of care. We can't pay the rent or mortgage, and they're also usually responsible for ensuring we're fed. However, beyond that, we are still responsible for many personal decisions. We are the only ones who can bathe or brush our own teeth, and it's our job to make sure we are picking the right foods and getting some healthy movement in.

Eating Right

Social media can contribute to disordered eating habits. What this means is eating in a way that doesn't promote a healthy relationship with food. One example of disordered eating is binge eating. This involves eating past the point of hunger. Usually, it involves eating mindlessly, without much thought. Binge eating can also be followed by periods of purging. Purging is either accomplished through periods of starvation or, in some cases, vomiting. Binging and purging are incredibly dangerous, especially to a developing teen's body. It can wreak havoc on your digestive system as well as your heart health. Healthy eating involves listening to your body and recognizing the different cues of hunger and feelings of fullness.

Seeing someone online with the perfect body can trigger the urge to participate in disordered eating. When you are feeling insecure about your appearance or inadequate, it's common to want to take drastic measures to achieve a certain body type.

You might feel the urge to skip meals as a way to starve yourself in order to fit into a certain body type. Alternatively, binge eating can help alleviate feelings of anxiety or depression temporarily. However, there is usually an extreme emotional crash involved after that period of eating, coupled with physical symptoms of overeating like nausea or stomachaches.

The effects that social media can have on a developing mind are very harmful, especially the mind of someone still growing and changing. As a teen, you are going to change so much over the next few years. There is no rush to get the perfect body, especially if it means potentially hurting your body's development. You already have the perfect body for you. We are all born with bodies that do their best to try and promote health. Some bodies look different than other bodies, and that is a truth of life that we will have to accept. What's important is ensuring that you provide your body with proper nutrition.

Often, eating is seen as a means to look a certain way, and over time, we lose sight of the real value of having healthy and nutritious meals, as the focus is placed on achieving a specific body type through our meals. It's easy to compare yourself to different bodies on social media, especially when certain body types are more likely to be promoted on social media apps like TikTok and Instagram. You will constantly see people wearing perfect clothing that accentuates certain body features. They have perfect skin and very few wrinkles. When you are constantly bombarded with specific body types all day, and then you look in the mirror and see that you don't have the same one, it can be very damaging to your self-esteem.

We also have to remember the lengths that people go to to achieve these certain body types including surgeries, injections, and other types of expensive or potentially damaging treatments. On top of that, many individuals have personal trainers and workouts to sculpt their bodies as a part of their everyday job. We simply do not have the same access to resources that those who are professional influencers or celebrities do.

As a teen, it's important for you to focus on intuitive eating. This means listening to your body and recognizing different hunger cues. Intuitive eating involves eating simply when you are hungry and stopping when you are full. There are many different hunger cues that you can listen to. The most obvious one is a grumbling stomach. We all know what it feels like when we are hungry. Beyond that, look for other signs in your body that it might be best to have a snack or eat a healthy meal. This involves things like having a headache or maybe even feeling nauseous or lightheaded.

When you're feeling stressed out or you find that you're having trouble focusing, this could also be a sign that you should consider eating something to help make you feel better.

It's also important to stop eating once you feel like you are full. If you do decide to eat even after you're full, then it's also important to let your body and mind know that this is okay. Attaching guilt and shame to your eating habits will only make it harder to follow a routine of healthy eating.

It's also important to focus on meals that are balanced. Balanced meals include a diverse range of foods from different food groups. This means eating healthy carbohydrates, vegetables, fruits, and protein sources. If you are going to be eating something like pizza, or greasy fried chicken, there's no shame in that. All food is good food if it makes you feel full. The important thing is to pair it with something nutritious as well. This might mean eating some sauteed spinach if you're going to have fried chicken or eating a side salad filled with tomatoes, onions, lettuce, and mixed greens. The most important thing to focus on in your developing years is balance, and to have a good relationship with food.

The guilt and shame that are attached to unhealthy eating habits can be just as damaging to your mental health as unhealthy eating is to your physical health. If you start repairing that relationship, you'll notice that it is easier to make healthier decisions for your body in the end.

Getting Movement

On top of healthy eating, it's important that we get enough physical exercise in our routine. Just like eating, exercise can often be associated with physical appearance. Exercise can give you certain aesthetic results, but the most important thing to focus on is exercising in order to help your body function properly. Exercising keeps everything moving through your systems. This means your digestive, neurological, and cardiovascular systems are all worked out through the various movements that you do with your body.

Social media contributes to a sedentary lifestyle, so it's essential that we incorporate more methods of healthy movement into our lives. It's recommended for teens to get at least one hour of physical activity daily (Mathe, 2022).

Exercise can be broken up into small parts throughout the day. While an hour might be recommended daily, it doesn't necessarily have to be consecutive. You might go for a 30-minute walk and then do small bits of 10-minute exercises three other times throughout the day.

If you're in a gym class, then you are likely already getting a good chunk of your workout in. There's pressure to go to the gym or exercise in a certain way, but you don't necessarily have to do that. Do small things like running up and down the stairs a few times in between study sessions. Stand up and do a few squats or push-ups against the wall. Try doing a wall sit while you are listening to an audiobook. Before you hop in the shower, consider doing some jumping jacks or another exercise that you can do in place. You don't have to go to the gym for three hours today to stay healthy. As long as you're moving your body consistently throughout the day and feeling a little bit of muscle strain, you will still be able to get some of the benefits of exercise.

The more regularly you make movement a part of your life, the easier it will be to do it throughout your adult life as well. Do more active things with friends. This means going on walks and jogs with them.

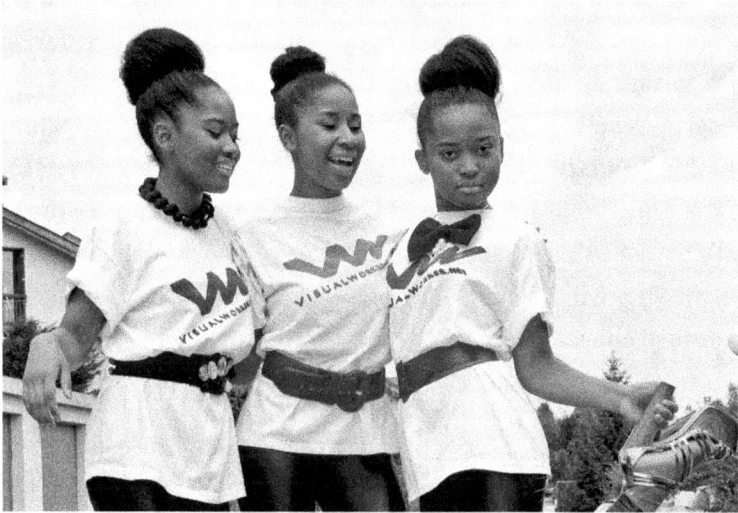

Go to your local nature walks or national parks in your state and explore nature with somebody else. Take your family dog on a walk. Play with them outside in the backyard. Come up with games with your friends, your pets, and your siblings. When you can make exercise a fun activity rather than something you feel pressured to do, you are more likely to participate in it. Dancing is also a great way to get more movement in. You can dance alone in your bedroom or you can dance with friends in social settings. Invest in some small forms of exercise equipment like resistance bands or even a stair stepper that you can do when listening to audiobooks or watching educational things so that you can multitask by getting in physical movement and learning at the same time.

Staying Hydrated

Sometimes we feel terrible simply because we have not drunk enough water!

Hydration is just as important as proper nutrition. Drinking enough water and staying hydrated throughout the day is important to help with digestion. It also helps with your energy levels. If you feel sick or tired, or you're struggling with a headache, try drinking a glass of water. It's powerful in helping you calm down, stay focused, and feel better over-all. Invest in a reusable water bottle so that you always have it on you. Most classrooms allow you to have water bottles because educators know the importance of staying hydrated.

Add more hydrating foods to your diet like lettuce, strawberries, watermelon, or peppers. Hydration isn't just absorbed through water but also through healthy foods. Try to aim for six to eight glasses of water a day and make sure that you sip them slowly and consistently. Chugging five glasses of water in a row is not going to give you the hydration that you need. This can also be very damaging to your internal organs as your kidneys and liver will have to filter that out and can become overwhelmed with the amount of water that you're drinking.

It's important to stay hydrated up until you go to bed and also ensure that you hydrate first thing in the morning. When you're sleeping for 10 hours, that's a long time for your body to go without water, so sip a glass of water slowly in the morning along with your breakfast. Drink water with every meal and every beverage that you have as well. Things like sugary soda and even diet sodas can be very dehydrating on the body, so it's important to drink water along with other beverages. Hydration is just one important part of maintaining your health overall.

Getting Sleep

One of the biggest contributing factors to a lack of sleep for teens is social media use. The CDC recommends that teens between 13 and 18 get between 8 and 10 hours of sleep per night ("Sleep," 2020).

When it comes to getting proper sleep, consistency is key. As mentioned previously, we all have a circadian rhythm. This is a pattern that naturally occurs in our body and helps to regulate our hormones. When getting proper sleep at night, it's important to stay consistent so that you can help maintain your body's natural rhythm. Try to wake up and go to sleep around the same time every day. This means that if you have to wake up at 6 a.m., it's important to be asleep by 10 p.m. the night before, or even 8 p.m. if you can swing it.

Some teens might see this and feel overwhelmed. They might believe there's no way that they could get that much sleep because they have schoolwork and after-school activities along with trying to maintain a social life. Napping is also helpful, so if you aren't able to get 8 hours of sleep a night, it's important to try and get a little nap in at some point in the day when you have the time. If you're feeling overwhelmed and like you're struggling with focusing, it might be because you're not getting enough sleep. Once you start to actually properly energize your body, you'll find that you're more productive and able to focus easier, therefore lightening your workload.

Make sure that you're falling asleep around the same time every night and not just getting into bed around that time. If you do have to fall asleep by 10 p.m. at night, try getting into bed by 9:30 p.m. so that you can give yourself plenty of time to fall asleep. You can also try catching up on sleep on the weekends. Just ensure that you aren't depending on this catch-up period. It's something to simply do on weeks when you might not have gotten proper sleep during the weekdays.

When it comes to using social media, it is incredibly important to not use it in your bed. Our minds have a sort of muscle memory where we get used to the habits that we have. This is why tying your shoes and brushing your teeth are both second nature. Our bodies store our activities so that they take less energy to participate in them. When you are getting into bed every night and reaching for your phone and scrolling on social media, this creates muscle memory that tells you that as soon as you get under the covers, you should probably reach for your phone. Break this habit by not using your phone in bed at all. You can still check up on social media before you go to bed. Just try doing it in the living room or another area of your home so that you don't have the muscle memory associated with late nights on social media. If you can, it's best to keep your phone in a different room altogether and use an external alarm clock. You might also have your parents wake you up if you don't want to rely on an alarm clock. When you can keep your phone outside of the room, you'll be much less likely to be up all night on social media.

If you have to sleep with a nightlight on because you don't like the dark, then make sure that you pick one that is timed and doesn't stay on all night. It's okay if you have a light on for 30 minutes as you're trying to fall asleep. Many people don't like complete pitch-black darkness. This is why many people also sleep with the television on. However, lights like this, especially ones that change throughout the night, are very disruptive to your sleep. Even if you are falling asleep, that TV on in the background might have some noise or flashing lights that keep you from reaching the really deep stages of sleep that you need for restoration. Put a timer on your TV or invest in a nightlight that has a timer so that it goes off within 30 minutes of you falling asleep. This way, you can be in the pitch-black darkness and able to reach those very crucial restoration stages at night.

When you are able to ensure that you're giving your body proper nutrition, hydration, physical movement, and sleep, you are connecting all the corners of your health, making it easier for you to stay focused and reduce feelings of stress, anxiety, and depression.

Proper Hygiene

When we feel down about ourselves, it's hard to keep up with our hygiene. Of course, styling hair and putting on clean clothes is often done for aesthetic reasons, but it can also change how we view ourselves in general.

The last thing to focus on when it comes to self-care is proper hygiene. Having clean hair, brushing your teeth, and getting dressed in the morning is something many of us do because we feel the pressure to do so. When it comes to weekends or days that you're not doing anything, you might not get dressed up. You might stay in your pajamas most of the day, or maybe you don't style your hair. You might skip the shower and avoid putting yourself together at all because it doesn't seem as important if you're not going to be seen by other people. However, hygiene is still something important to participate in every day, beyond just for reasons associated with the way that we look. We need to focus on the way that it makes us *feel*.

Getting dressed and out of your pajamas is important so that you feel more prepared for the day. Brushing your teeth and washing your hair is a way to cleanse yourself and feel like a new person. You can wash the day away in a hot bath or shower. Brushing your teeth gives you a more refreshing feeling, and doing things like washing your face and maintaining your fingernails can make you feel more confident, even when you aren't seeing other people. It's important for us to separate the pressure of participating in hygiene based on the way that we look and instead rework our relationship with it so that we can focus on taking care of ourselves and making ourselves feel like our best versions.

Follow the tips below to help you maintain your hygiene:

- Shower daily. Whether you want to shower when you wake up in the morning or shower before you go to bed at night, that is completely up to you. Daily showers help us to wash away potentially harmful bacteria while also feeling refreshed. You don't have to wash your hair every day. You can wash your hair two to three times a week. However, a quick, brisk shower can be very rejuvenating. Make sure that you clean every part of your body from the top of your head to the tips of your toes. Use a loofah to help really scrub away some of those dead skin cells and make sure that the soap is very lathered.

- Brush your teeth twice a day. If you forget or you only decide to brush once a day, then it's more important to brush at night before you go to bed, as this helps ensure that you don't have food and sugar sitting on your teeth all night while you're sleeping. However, brushing twice a day is incredibly important because bacteria can form in our mouths overnight, especially when sleeping with our mouths open. As such, brushing your teeth in the morning is just as important as at night. Make sure that you're also scraping your tongue. Having good tongue hygiene is good for maintaining clean and fresh breath.

- Make sure to style or at least attend to your hair daily. This means brushing it, combing it, or tying it back. Make sure that you get rid of the knots that are in it. When you do wash your hair, make sure to focus on your scalp and wash away the dirt and oil there. Don't overlook your nails when maintaining proper hygiene. A lot of bacteria can get trapped under your fingernails, especially if you have really long fingernails. Keep them trimmed. This will also help you avoid biting your nails if you find that you're somebody who has issues with biting and picking.

- Lastly, don't overlook skincare. Even though you are youthful and have plenty of natural restorative processes in your skin, it's still helpful to make sure that you're washing your face daily to keep acne at bay and moisturize so that you feel like your best self.

Reminders

- **Step #5**: Take care of yourself.

You only have one mind, one body, and one life to live. Whenever you run into something online that makes you feel inadequate or like you are not good enough, remember to stay grounded in reality. Check the facts. Who posted this? Is there any way that this could be edited or inflated to look better than reality? What is the intention behind what is being posted? Social media can be heavily influential over our mindset, so it's important to stay proactive about caring for your mental health as you navigate the online world through your teenage years.

6. Replace Old Habits

The urge to constantly check our phone is deeply embedded in our psyche because it's a habit, so understanding how to break apart a habit will enable you to turn it into something more useful.

Many people have bad habits that are hard to break, like procrastinating. However, procrastination isn't necessarily something everyone does. Those who do procrastinate are usually alone when they are doing it. When we use our phones excessively, we do it consistently and out in the open. We do it in settings where everyone can see, and phone use is normalized. For this reason, it can be hard to notice when a habit is turning into something that is destructive to your life. Raising awareness is the first step in breaking a habit.

The Power of Mindfulness

The pressure to reach for our phones often happens automatically and without much thought. By encouraging a stronger sense of mindfulness on a day-to-day basis, we will be able to stay one step ahead of these impulses.

What Is Mindfulness?

Mindfulness is a powerful tool that has been known to decrease anxiety and depression, as well as other health issues like sleep disorders, excess stress, and chronic pain (Mandriota, 2022).

Mindfulness is a mental process that helps ground you in the moment. When we are struggling with anxiety, depression, or other forms of unwanted emotions, we can use mindfulness as a tool to keep us in the present. This involves noticing your sensations and raising bodily and spatial awareness. Why is it important to be mindful? If we are not mindful, then we lose sight of reality. We get stuck in our own thought process. If you are somebody who struggles with social anxiety, for example, then you will end up getting stuck in your own head. You will start to replay past scenarios and see them in a darker, more anxiety-inducing way. You will start to go over a situation that you've already lived through and feel very negatively about it. You might hyper-fixate on all of the little things that you said while overlooking the reality, which is that most people aren't as fixated on the little things you said as you are.

Our phones also strip us of the ability to be mindful because they transport us to another world. Not only do they provide a distraction, but they also bring up unwanted emotions that are easy to ruminate on. Rumination is the process of going over the same thoughts or feelings in your head repeatedly.

Most of us know that people edit their pictures, so we shouldn't make comparisons to what we see online. However, in reality, many of us still end up struggling with comparison and ultimately feeling bad about ourselves, even though we know deep down we shouldn't be making these types of comparisons. Increasing mindfulness means we are more present in the here and now, therefore, we have more control over our thoughts and actions. You can use mindfulness when you're stressed about life in general, or feeling triggered by social media.

Right now, grab something small that's sitting next to you. Whether it's a lip balm, a coin, a pencil, or something else small, hold it in your hand and get a sense of how it feels. Notice the textures and the sensation that it has in your hand as you're holding it. Trace your finger along the outside edge of this object. Notice the way that your thoughts might be trying to convert back to anxiety as you're doing this. You might still feel that anxious feeling deep in your stomach and in your core, and it can be hard to look past. However, as long as you keep focusing on this object here and now in the present moment, then eventually those anxious feelings will dissipate. Below are a few more examples of mindfulness activities we can participate in to help reduce anxiety and increase presence in the moment.

Five Senses

One mindfulness activity to participate in is the five senses activity. Most of us have five senses. These include the ability to see hear, touch, taste, and smell. When you are feeling anxious, it's important to notice all these sensations. The five senses activity is as follows:

1. First, identify five things in the room that you can see. What is around you? What shapes do you notice? What colors do you notice? What objects are around you? What people or animals are in the room with you? Where are you? What place are you in? What setting are you in? Identify all these different types of things.
2. Second, notice four things that you can touch. This includes the chair you're sitting in, the cushions that you're using, and the texture of the clothes that you're wearing. What do you feel under your feet? What do you feel with your hands? What do you feel with your entire body? Notice four things that you can use to help you feel connected to your touch sense.
3. Third, pay attention to three things that you can hear. Do you hear the air conditioning or heating system running? Do you hear birds or animals outside? Do you hear kids playing? Do you hear somebody talking in the next room? Do you hear your own feet fidgeting around underneath you? What three things are in the room that make noises?
4. Identify two things that you can smell. Do you smell an air freshener? Do you smell food cooking in the

other room? What kinds of scents are surrounding you at this moment? If you can't identify any smell, then you can identify the sense through certain objects in the room that might have a scent. For example, if you see a picture of flowers hanging on the wall, try to visualize the scent of the flowers. If you see an unopened bag of chips sitting across the room, think about the smell of the chips.

5. Lastly, identify one thing that you can taste. The same thing might happen with your taste sense where you can't identify something that holds an actual flavor, but try to identify objects that you can associate with this sense. For example, if you're sitting in the doctor's office waiting room feeling anxious, there might not really be anything around that has a flavor. However, there is still likely something that you can visualize the taste of. If you see the sign for the bathroom, think about water coming from the faucet, and think about the taste of water. It's also helpful if you carry mints on you so that you can actually physically taste something at the moment to keep yourself more present. Even if you can't visualize something actually edible, consider the taste of things around you. What might the wall taste like? What might the carpet taste like? It seems really silly to think about, but it's still a way that you can stay more focused at the moment and help your thoughts get distracted from a place of anxiety and instead focus on the present.

Identifying your five senses is a way to ground you in the present and make you more aware of some of the bodily sensations that you are experiencing.

Color Identification

The second mindfulness activity is the color identification one. This involves looking around you and identifying all of the objects in a room that are specific colors. Let's try it right now. Consider the color yellow. This is a very common color. How many objects do you see in the room with you that are yellow? Perhaps this is a book or a throw pillow. Maybe there's a yellow candle or something yellow in the portrait hanging on the wall. This feels like a really simple activity, but it can be enough to bring you into the present moment so that you stop ruminating over some of your thoughts and anxieties. Try going through the rainbow and identifying everything in the room that's red, orange, yellow, green, blue, and purple. Then, identify the colors that aren't in the rainbow like black, gray, pink, and white. Once you have gone through all of these types of colors, you'll likely find that your thoughts have stopped ruminating and cycling through your anxieties and it's easier for you to stay present in the moment.

Take it a step further and identify different textures or materials. What in the room is made out of wood? How many objects can you identify that are made out of metal? Do you notice any plants? Consider anything soft or fuzzy. Paying attention to these types of spatial elements brings you back into the present moment. This is something really important to do, especially after we use our phones to scroll through social media. Once you hit close on your phone and set it down, take a moment to be mindful and pull yourself back into the present. It's really easy to see something triggering online or to be struggling with your thoughts and let that spiral. This thought spiral can end up affecting your behavior and what actions you take next, so it's crucial that we stay present in the moment after using our phones.

Body Scan

The last mindfulness activity to try is a body scan. This will help you connect with your body and really feel better and more present in the moment. Social media is something that happens first mentally. We stare at our phones and we think all these thoughts that come along and are triggered by our cell phone usage. It's crucial that you connect back to your body so that you can become more aware of all the ways that you're feeling. A body scan involves literally scanning our body by using our minds from the top of our heads down to the bottom of our feet. To do a body scan, take a moment and focus on each part of your body while taking deep breaths. This means starting on your head and taking a big, deep breath in. Hold it for a moment and then slowly let it out.

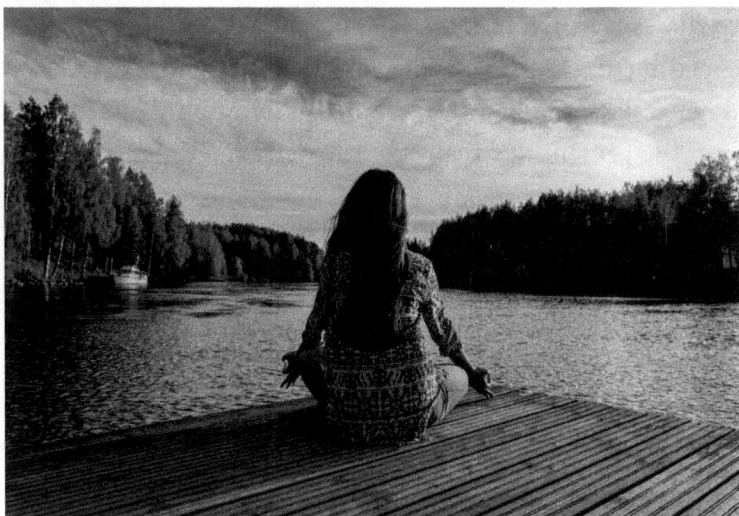

Pay attention to your head and everything on it. Notice your forehead, your eyebrows, your nose, your eyes, your cheeks, your tongue, your lips, your chin, your ears, the back of your neck, and so on. Scan down to your torso next. Notice your arms, your elbows, your fingertips, your wrists, your chest, your belly button, your abdomen, and your hips. Lastly, focus on your legs. Think about your butt, your thighs, your knees, the back of your knees, your calves, your shins, your ankles, your feet, your heel, and your toes.

Once you scan from the top to the bottom, scan again from the bottom to the top, each time taking a moment and lingering on that specific body part as you deeply breathe in and out. You can also pair this with muscle relaxation. This involves tensing the muscle that you're focusing on and then releasing it before moving on. If you pair this with deep breathing, you will find that your anxiety decreases instantly, and the more that you repeat this practice, the easier it will be to have mindfulness become an active part of your life.

Exploring Your Passions

With all of the free time and motivation you have after reducing screen time, it's important to discover greater passions in life. Passions are good for taking up free time and providing you with value, and there's science behind that. Studies prove teens who find their passion are less likely to participate in "risky behavior," including things like drugs, crime, and sex ("How and Why," 2016).

Some research also suggests that finding a passion is better for your future than trying to choose a career due to the consistent changes in the job field (Bridges, n.d.). If you are able to be more mindful of what you actually want to do versus what you feel pressured to do, it will be much easier to carve out time to explore your passions.

Growth Mindset

During your teenage years and even as a young adult, your brain is going to continue to develop. During these times of brain development, it's important to focus on fostering a growth mindset. What does it mean to have a growth mindset? To understand this, let's first start by discussing what a fixed mindset is.

A fixed mindset is one that follows the same types of thinking patterns without stepping outside of the box. When it comes to solving problems, there are usually multiple different types of solutions that you can utilize to help you resolve an issue. A fixed mindset is one that only sees life in one singular way. Indeed, a fixed mindset is one that follows everything that it has been taught without questioning some of these rules and regulations.

One thing a fixed mindset does is follow cognitive distortions. A cognitive distortion is a pattern of thinking that can lead to bad or unpleasant emotions. Cognitive refers to the way that we use our brain and how our thoughts develop to shape our actions. A cognitive distortion is a pattern of thinking that is a little more unhealthy.

Think of it like eating chips versus eating carrots. Both are foods. Both are things you shouldn't feel guilty about eating or not eating. However, if you only ever eat chips and never eat carrots (or other vegetables), then you might end up feeling sick and unwell. A cognitive distortion is a pattern of thinking that will always keep us feeling very sad. While everyone has cognitive distortions from time to time (like chips), too many of these thought patterns can hurt your health.

One type of cognitive distortion is black-and-white thinking. This is when you see a situation as being either entirely good or entirely bad. Sometimes we try to put things into specific boxes and make categorizations to help us understand their meaning. For example, some people might think if you are good at sports, maybe that means you're not very good at schoolwork. Other people might think if you are good at schoolwork and you love reading, you're not going to be as athletically talented. Black-and-white thinking can take the shape of more "traditional" thinking as well. For example, you might assume that when you go to see a doctor, it's going to be male. Despite the fact that the medical industry is filled with intelligent women, if you think traditionally, you might associate certain positions with gender. Think of construction workers. You might assume that one is going to be a man. However, there are plenty of female construction workers. When you think of a stay-at-home parent who cares for the children, black-and-white thinking might lead you to believe that this is usually a mother. However, a more open mindset can help you see that no specific role is attached to a specific person. This is just one example of how we might get stuck in our thoughts and fail to see all of the other complex and realistic situations that exist.

Another type of cognitive distortion is personalization. This refers to when you might assume that a situation is about you. If you are walking by a group of people and you hear them laugh, you might think to yourself that they're making fun of you, or that they're laughing because they're teasing you. In reality, they're just laughing about something funny that happened earlier, or maybe one of their friends in the group shared a joke. Personalization can make us feel as though the world is out to get us and that we are very isolated from other people. It can make us feel really insecure and scared to be ourselves. Another example of personalization is how we might feel embarrassed after social situations. If you are to go to a friend's party, you might say something silly or maybe you even do something a little embarrassing, like spill your soda. After the party, you go home and feel really embarrassed about that small moment. Even though it was only a few minutes, you still can't help but think that it ruined the entirety of the party. In reality, most of the people forgot about what happened and they were more focused on their own embarrassing moments as well.

A growth mindset is a way that we can utilize mental challenges and obstacles to explore new parts of our brain. After you walk by that group of snickering people, rather than thinking to yourself, *Oh, they must be laughing at me*, instead, you can challenge that thought and think, *Actually, they're probably just laughing at something else.*

One way to help foster a growth mindset is to try new things and explore areas that you maybe thought you didn't like. Social media makes it easy to cater our worldview into something that serves us and revolves around the specific things that we like. It's easy to create a box that you feel safe inside of, and you might only surround yourself with the things that you and your friends like. However, when we follow the same ways of thinking over and over again, that can eventually lead to cognitive distortions. It's important to break free from this box and think in new ways to reduce feelings of anxiety and depression.

Hobbies to Try

To help you keep exploring your passions and the things that you like, it's essential that you try many different hobbies. Hobbies are great things to help fill the time that you have once you start to detox from excessive social media use. Let's discuss a few different categories of hobbies that you can try to help you foster a new mindset.

The first is crafts. Consider artistic crafts that you can do on your own. These include things like knitting or sewing. These are great things to do while you are listening to an audiobook, watching TV, or even hanging out with friends. Crafts like these help keep your hands busy so that you're less likely to reach for your phone. Continue exploring your creativity through other artistic hobbies like drawing, painting, or pottery. All of these types of artistic hobbies let you explore different parts of your brain. Whenever you are creating something, you have to think of an idea and then you have to actually execute that idea. After you're done with the creation, you have to look at what you made and evaluate it. You can see the things that you like, which makes you feel good about yourself. You can also see areas of improvement, helping you to build your skills so that you are even more talented the next time around. You can also try other crafts like woodworking.

Aside from creative hobbies, consider different hobbies that involve nature. This includes gardening, horticulture, or environmentalism. Head to your local library and check out books on birds in your area, or trees in your area, and walk around your neighborhood to see how many different varieties you can identify.

Lastly, it's important to explore literature outside of an educational context. This means having a relationship with books and writing that doesn't involve schoolwork. Academics can make us feel very pressured to read and write in a certain way. When you are forced to read assignments and work on different papers, it can make you feel really disconnected from the act of reading and writing. However, both of these skills are very important not just for your professional life in the future, but also to help you explore your mind and grow your knowledge. Find different books of genres that you like. Consider young adult, horror, or science fiction novels. You can also explore nonfiction books in areas that you are interested in. Writing is also important to try outside of school. When you don't have the pressure of getting graded for what you're writing, it's easier for you to explore your mindset and let your words flow freely.

Lastly, consider volunteering. Volunteering is a great way to help you build up your experience. Find volunteer work in your area, especially in subjects that you feel passionate about. This might mean heading to your local animal shelter to help volunteer by taking care of the animals. Perhaps you can volunteer through the park district to help keep nature clean. You can volunteer through your school or local sports if you are an athletic person who wants to work with a specific sport more frequently. Volunteering not only looks good on a future job application or college application, but it's also a great way to meet new people and stay connected. When you fill your free time with hobbies, volunteer work, and other activities, you are less likely to spend excessive amounts of time on social media.

Reminders

- **Step #6**: Increase mindfulness to reduce social media habits.

Our phones are like new limbs in modern society. They are there first thing in the morning and we often check them right before bed at night. We rarely leave the house without them and we make sure to check in with them multiple times throughout the day. The best way to ensure we are staying aware of social media use is through the act of mindfulness. Phone use isn't all bad, so learning how to utilize mindfulness with it will ensure you can maintain a healthy relationship with social media.

7. Repair Your Relationship

Social media doesn't have to be entirely demonized and banished from one's life in order to have beneficial results. Rather, rebuilding a stronger relationship with it will help you thrive in the future without perpetuating an all-or-nothing mindset.

An all-or-nothing mindset is another cognitive distortion. This means that you either have to use *all* of something or none of it at all. For example, dieting can perpetuate an all-or-nothing mindset. Some believe that if they have just one slice of cake or one piece of candy, then they've broken their "diet," therefore they should just give up on healthy eating altogether. That's not the case at all! It's fine to focus on healthy foods while still enjoying a treat every now and then.

Social media isn't something to approach with an all-or-nothing mindset. You can still enjoy it in a healthy way without feeling like you have to give it up altogether.

The Healthy Benefits of Social Media

Social media is much like a tool, and tools can either be used to destroy things or build something amazing. Knowing how to use social media to your advantage will ensure that you maintain a healthy relationship with it.

Most of the adverse effects of social media reported through studies and research are associated with a high amount of use as well as the type of content viewed (Cullen, 2023). If you are able to reduce how much you are using it while focusing on more positive aspects of social media, you will then be able to take advantage of the benefits rather than suffering from the negative effects.

Stay Connected

Over half of teens reported that social media was actually beneficial to their friendships according to one study, and around a third believed it improved confidence (Gordon, 2022).

The reason social media was invented in the first place was to help us stay connected to other people. This was established so that we could reach out to others and share our interests online. Socialization can be difficult for some. Finding a place to meet up with other people and actually taking the time out of your day to get ready and go out and chat with others can be very tiring. It's easy for us to isolate, especially when we live in areas where it's not easy to get together with other people. If you live in a very rural area and don't have access to transportation, you might find that you spend a lot of time at home, not necessarily by choice, but because you don't have many other options. Social media is a great way for us to stay connected and to feel more close to other people. We can meet new people and we can chat with them whenever we want.

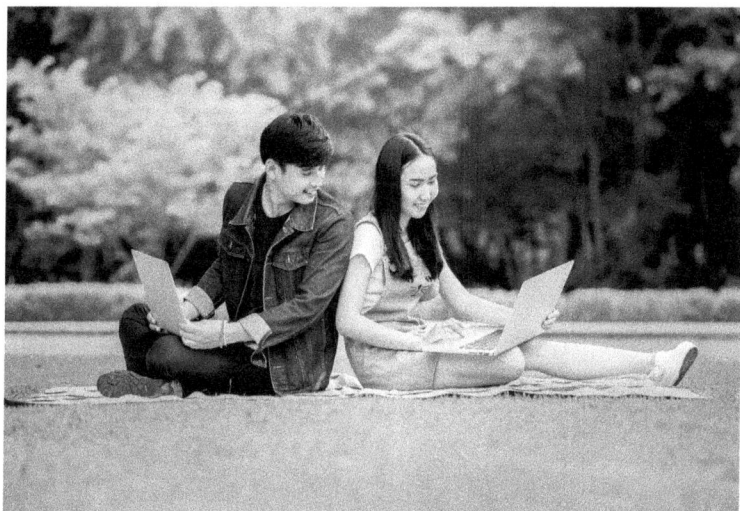

You are no longer limited to just the people in your area either. You can connect to people across the world. Social media is a great and powerful tool that you can use to stay connected; you simply have to know how to use it. One important thing to do is to ensure that you cut out those who are toxic and bring you down. Instead, focus on filling your online presence with those who inspire you and lift you up. It's okay to unfollow people who you're not friends with. One good rule is that if you wouldn't approach them in public to have a conversation, then you shouldn't follow them online. Sometimes we see people who we simply have curiosities about. It's not necessarily that you like that person or that you're friends with them, you might just follow them because you're in an athletic activity together or because you both go to the same school. You don't need to stay connected to these people if they make you feel self-conscious, insecure, or like you are not good enough.

When you cut out people who you're not that interested in, it also provides you with the freedom to express yourself, making connections even easier. If you have 2,000 followers and you only know 20 of them personally, then when you post online, you're curating your presence to people you don't even know. This can lead you to feel pressured to make specific posts and present your life in a certain way, which can add a lot of stress and anxiety to your social media use. When you have a small network of people following you, it's much easier to post things that you actually care about, therefore making it easier for others to reach out and stay connected.

Professional Development

Consider using social media for professional development. This is a great way to create a professional network and stay connected to those who could potentially help us in our careers. This might mean staying connected to certain teachers or other educational individuals in your life. You can stay connected with people so that you can ask for letters of recommendation later in life. You can also stay connected so that you can share different parts of your work and maintain aspects of career development.

Consider having a strictly professional social media that you can develop over time and use to get a head start in your career. When you're posting things, you can use hashtags to help you connect with other professionals in the area. When you create a network of people who could help you professionally in the future, social media becomes an excellent resource to have. This means connecting with people who can provide you with job opportunities, or at least inspire you within your career.

We don't have to know exactly what we want to do with our lives as teens, but if you start a professional social media account, it can help you get a greater sense of what area you might be interested in exploring. For example, if you're really passionate about writing, you can start a writing-specific account where you share your work and connect to other writers. You might be very business-minded and you want to open up a business in the future. You can connect with people who inspire you and create a network of role models so that you are exposed to valuable insight. You might be very passionate about cooking and one day you want to open your own restaurant or even have your own cooking show. There are plenty of resources online for you to connect with others, helping you to build a strong portfolio and social media presence over time.

Learning Opportunities

Social media is great for endless amounts of learning opportunities. We just have to ensure that we are following the right people who are educated on these topics. For example, one great learning opportunity through social media is social justice issues. You might be interested in learning about inequalities between different demographics. You might be a passionate environmentalist, so you can connect with activists in your area to learn about how you might be able to help. You can follow educational pages and those that provide realistic and practical tips. Just ensure when you do this, you know the ins and outs of fact-checking and you're able to find sources to back up what people are sharing. You can do this for career purposes, or you can simply do it to help fill your free time. You can follow science pages that share interesting information, or entertainment pages that share interesting facts about your favorite shows and movies. There are endless amounts of learning opportunities on social media, so if you start curating your online presence around this, then you'll be getting fed even more types of educational pages, therefore crafting a perfect algorithm of helpful resources rather than one that makes you feel bad about yourself.

Keeping Addictions at Bay

Knowing the benefits of social media will keep you focused on creating a productive and helpful online presence. When you are focused on mindfulness and using social media in the right way, it's easier to keep addictions at bay. However, because social media can be so addictive and habitual, it's easy to fall back into old ways. Below are a few more tips to help you manage social media use.

Make Anonymous Profiles

One tip to help you navigate social media is to make anonymous profiles. Consider creating a separate account outside of who you know in your personal life. This way, you can use social media without the pressure to create a certain image online. You can simply have an Instagram account where you follow different meme pages or other profiles and follow people who you're interested in, without the pressure to post or have a presence yourself. You can use social media as a way to watch others and entertain yourself without feeling the urge to perfectly curate an image. You can simply log on and use social media in whatever way you want without anybody knowing what you're doing online. Sometimes we feel hesitant to follow certain people or to share certain posts because of what others might think. When you remove other people from your social media use, you can then just simply enjoy it for what it is. This also helps protect your privacy.

Another important tip is to avoid liking or saving things on social media. Liking can also add a lot of pressure and can be a part of your image. Some people simply like everything. It doesn't matter who posted it, or what the post actually is. If it's somebody that they follow, they might simply like that post. Other people might feel a lot of pressure about what to like. You might even have a time in your past when you liked a post and then decided to go back later and unlike it. It's good to have a rule to simply not like anything at all.

The same can be said for saving different things online. For example, if you are constantly saving videos that you want to go back and watch later, chances are you likely won't end up watching them later. Keep your social media clutter-free just in the way that you would your home. This can help reduce feelings of being overwhelmed and other pressures that social media can bring on.

Use Other Social Media

Going forward, consider changing the types of social media that you use altogether. What platforms do you currently have an account on? Chances are you likely have a TikTok, YouTube, or Instagram account. Consider deactivating or even deleting some of these and instead creating new types of social media. For example, you might create an account on something like Goodreads or Letterboxed. These are websites that can help you track different movies or books that you read and watch. This is a great way to stay connected to other people and also help you develop some of your interests. You can still log on to see what people are up to without the pressure of posting your body or other aspects of your lifestyle. You can still have some insight into what others are interested in without the anxiety and stress that can come along and have a perfectly curated image. There are many different types of social media that are specific to the interests that we have. If you find one that fits what you are passionate about, consider focusing on this as your main social media.

Screen-Free Day

To help you keep up with healthy social media use in the future, consider having a screen-free day every single week. Screen-free Saturday has a nice ring to it, don't you think? Perhaps you want to do screen-free Sunday. These can be self-care days so that you can focus on doing things that make you feel good about yourself rather than spending excessive amounts of time on social media. Not only will this help you cut back on unhealthy use, but you will be even more aware of your use later on. In addition, you can also increase gratitude over social media use on the days that you are actually using it. For example, if you go every Saturday without social media, then when Sunday comes around, you might be more appreciative of it since you went without it for 24 hours.

Having a screen-free day every week is a perfect way to ensure that you keep any potential addictions at bay. You can still use social media throughout the rest of the week. What you will find is that having one day to set aside for productivity will make every other day of that week feel even better. You can use social media without feeling guilty or like you are doing it too much. Consider this challenge for at least a month. That means you only have to go four days without social media in a month! What you might find is that you feel so much better that you want to do multiple screen-free days a week. Whatever you decide to do with your free time is completely up to you. The most important thing to remember is to pay attention to how you're using social media and then how it makes you feel. Staying mindful and creating a level of awareness with social media use will ensure that you make the most of it without feeling the many negative side effects that could come along with excessive screen time.

Reminders

- **Step #7**: Rework your relationship with social media to use it for good.

Social media is here to stay, and it's not going away anytime soon. For some, it's how they met their partners. For others, it's how they make a career. As long as you focus on using it to your advantage, you will be able to free yourself from the restraints of addiction to live a more mindful and peaceful life.

Conclusion

Can you remember the first time you got on social media? For many, it's become such an ingrained part of our lives that it's hard to remember life without it.

Going forward, it's important to remember that social media doesn't have to be a bad thing. The main focus should be on how it makes you feel rather than giving in to the pressures that it can create.

Remember to follow the seven steps laid out throughout the book to help you on your social media detox journey:

1. Understand the impact that social media can have on your life. We're glued to our phones, so lacking awareness can mean failing to realize just how much stress and anxiety it can cause.
2. Recognize the dangers social media has had on your life. Social media is filled with funny videos and goofy memes, so it's easy to lose sight of how

dangerous and damaging it can be to our privacy and personal lives.

3. Reduce how much time you spend on your phone. The best way to start changing social media habits for the better is to incorporate small ways to reduce phone usage over time.

4. Take some time away from social media. Doing a total detox will help you realize just how dependent you are on this habit, while simultaneously freeing up your time so you can focus on the things you're interested in.

5. Take care of yourself. The intense emotions that social media brings can lead us to neglect our health and our needs, so remember to focus on self-care going forward.

6. Increase mindfulness to reduce social media habits. Raising awareness of the present moment will make you less inclined to mindlessly use social media.

7. Rework your relationship with social media to use it for good. Don't think of social media as a bad thing or feel like it should be demonized, as there are many benefits to gain from it.

There's no telling what your personal life will look like in the next decade, and most of us can't even fathom what the future holds for technology and social media. The best way to stay one step ahead of the hold your phone can have on you is to decrease use and maintain awareness in the present moment.

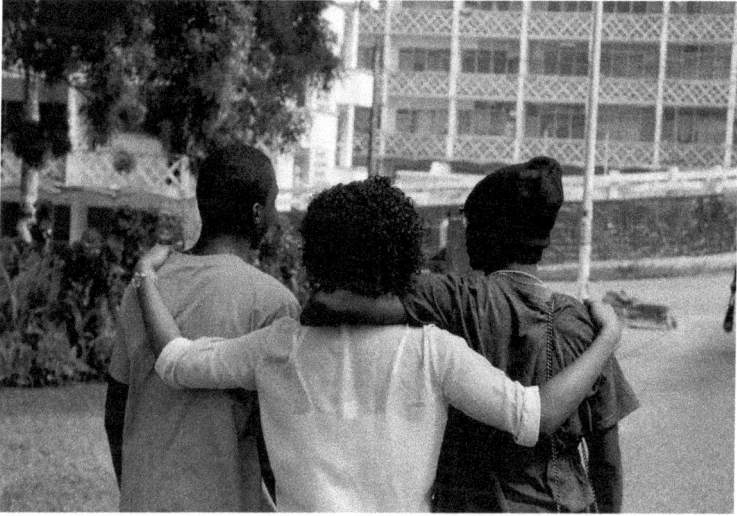

You only have one life to live, but the internet will be around forever. Taking care of yourself is the best way to ensure you're taking good care of your future.

References

Advertising: how it influences children and teenagers. (2022, December 10). Raising Children. https://raisingchildren.net.au/toddlers/play-learning/screen-time-media/advertising-children

Anderson, M., Perrin, A., Rainie, L., & Vogels, E. (2022, November 16). *Connection, creativity and drama: teen life on social media in 2022.* Pew Research Center. https://www.pewresearch.org/internet/2022/11/16/connection-creativity-and-drama-teen-life-on-social-media-in-2022/

Are you addicted to social media? (n.d.). Lee Health. https://www.leehealth.org/health-and-wellness/healthy-news-blog/mental-health/are-you-addicted-to-social-media

Bergman, M. (2023, September 18). *Social media's effects on self-esteem.* Social Media Victims Law Center. https://socialmediavictims.org/mental-health/self-esteem/

Bridges, C. (n.d.). *5 research-backed techniques to help teens develop passion.* Hello World. https://www.helloworldnetwork.org/post/5-research-backed-techniques-to-help-teens-develop-passion

Cassell, D. (2020, November 13). *Feeling more stress and anxiety? Your smartphone may be to blame.* Healthline. https://www.healthline.com/health-news/feeling-more-stress-and-anxiety-your-smartphone-may-be-to-blame

Chapman, S., Eyre, H., Keller, A., & MacRae, I. (2021, December 5). *Social media is changing our brains. Center for Brain Health.* https://centerforbrainhealth.org/article/social-media-is-changing-our-brains

Clifton, T. (2022, April 13). *Exercise for teenagers: A complete guide.* Healthline. https://www.healthline.com/health/fitness/exercise-for-teenagers

Cullen, K. (2023, January 28). *How to use social media without losing your mind.* Psychology Today. https://www.psychologytoday.com/us/blog/the-truth-about-exercise-addiction/202301/how-to-use-social-media-without-losing-your-mind

D'Onfro, J. (2018, January 10). *These simple steps will help you stop checking your phone so much.* CNBC. https://www.cnbc.com/2018/01/03/how-to-curb-you-smartphone-addiction-in-2018.html

Fotuhi, M. (2020, September 21). *What social media does to your brain.*

NeuroGrow. https://neurogrow.com/what-social-media-does-to-your-brain/

Gelles-Watnick, R. & Vogels, E. (2023, April 24). *Teens and social media: key findings from Pew Research Center surveys.* Pew Research Center. https://www.pewresearch.org/short-reads/2023/04/24/teens-and-social-media-key-findings-from-pew-research-center-surveys/

Gelles-Watnick, R., Massarat, N., & Vogels, E. (2022, August 10). *Teens, social media, and technology 2022.* Pew Research Center. https://www.pewresearch.org/internet/2022/08/10/teens-social-media-and-technology-2022/

Goldman, B. (2021, October 29). *Addictive potential of social media, explained.* Stanford Medicine. https://scopeblog.stanford.edu/2021/10/29/addictive-potential-of-social-media-explained/

Gordon, S. (2022, November 2). *Surprising ways your teen benefits from social media.* Verywell Family. https://www.verywellfamily.com/benefits-of-social-media-4067431

Green, M. (2023, January 9). *10 tips for a social media detox.* Pickard Properties. https://pickardproperties.co.uk/talking-points/10-tips-for-a-social-media-detox/

Health advisory on social media use in adolescence. (n.d.). American Psychological Association. https://www.apa.org/topics/social-media-internet/health-advisory-adolescent-social-media-use

Healthy social media habits. (2022, September). NIH. https://newsinhealth.nih.gov/2022/09/healthy-social-media-habits

Holmquist, J. (n.d.). *Social networking sites: consider the benefits, concerns for your teenager.* ICI. https://publications.ici.umn.edu/impact/24-1/social-networking-sites-consider-the-benefits-concerns-for-your-teenager

Horwood, S. (2022, December 11). *Constant smartphone notifications tax your brain.* Neuroscience News. https://neurosciencenews.com/smartphone-notifications-cognition-22048/

How and why teens should discover their passion. (2016, February 22). Middle Earth. https://middleearthnj.org/2016/02/22/how-and-why-teens-should-discover-their-passion/

Is your phone affecting your mental health? (2022, January 14). Butler Hospital. https://www.butler.org/blog/phone-affecting-your-mental-health

Keach, S. (2018, October 16). *Instagram tracks how much time you spend gawping at people's pics – and there's a good reason why.* The Sun. https://www.thesun.co.uk/tech/7508508/instagram-time-spent-photos-looking-stalking/

Lightman, A. (2021, January 15). *Teens have never known a world without data sharing, and it's creating a false sense of security.* NBC. https://www.nbcnews.com/think/opinion/teens-have-never-known-world-without-data-sharing-it-s-ncna1254332

Malouff, J. (2023, May 29). *What are the long-term effects of quitting social media? Almost nobody can log off long enough to find out.* The Conversation. https://theconversation.com/what-are-the-long-term-effects-of-quitting-social-media-almost-nobody-can-log-off-long-enough-to-find-out-205478

Miller, S. (2022, June 2). *The addictiveness of social media: how teens get hooked.* Jefferson Health. https://www.jeffersonhealth.org/your-health/living-well/the-addictiveness-of-social-media-how-teens-get-hooked

Millions of teenagers worry about body image and identify social media as a key cause – new survey by the Mental Health Foundation. (2019, May 15). Mental Health Foundation. https://www.mentalhealth.org.uk/about-us/news/millions-teenagers-worry-about-body-image-and-identify-social-media-key-cause-new-survey-mental

Morin, A. (2022, January 6). *How exposure to the media can harm your teen's body image.* Verywell Family. https://www.verywellfamily.com/media-and-teens-body-image-2611245

Ortiz, C. (2022, June 30). *7 mindfulness exercises for teens and tips to get started.* Psych Central. https://psychcentral.com/health/the-benefits-of-mindfulness-meditation-for-teens

Quinn, D. (2023, May 17). *Social media addiction: 4+ signs you're addicted to social media.* Sandstone Care. https://www.sandstonecare.com/blog/social-media-addiction/

Rogers, K. (2019, October 29). *US teens use screens more than seven hours a day on average – and that's not including school work.* CNN. https://www.cnn.com/2019/10/29/health/common-sense-kids-media-use-report-wellness/index.html

Schubert, A. (2021, March 30). *13 things that could happen when you quit social media.* The Healthy. https://www.thehealthy.com/mental-health/quit-social-media/

Sleep in middle and high school students. (2020, September 10). CDC. https://www.cdc.gov/healthyschools/features/students-sleep.htm

Smith, K. (2022, October 21). *6 common triggers of teen stress.* Psycom. https://www.psycom.net/common-triggers-teen-stress

Social media and teens. (2018, March). American Academy of Child & Adolescent Psychiatry. https://www.

aacap.org/AACAP/Families_and_Youth/Facts_for_Families/FFF-Guide/Social-Media-and-Teens-100.aspx

Staloch, L. (2023, February 4). *Exposure to social media can increase adolescent materialism but can be tempered with high self-esteem and mindfulness.* PsyPost. https://www.psypost.org/2023/02/exposure-to-social-media-can-increase-adolescent-materialism-but-can-be-tempered-with-high-self-esteem-and-mindfulness-67557

Strasburger, V. (2006). *Children, adolescents, and advertising.* American Academy of Pediatrics. https://publications.aap.org/pediatrics/article/118/6/2563/69735/Children-Adolescents-and-Advertising?autologincheck=redirected

Study shows habitual checking of social media may impact young adolescents' brain development. (2023, January 3). The University of North Carolina at Chapel Hill. https://www.unc.edu/posts/2023/01/03/study-shows-habitual-checking-of-social-media-may-impact-young-adolescents-brain-development/

Summer, J. (2023, October 12). *How blue light affects kids' sleep.* Sleep Foundation. https://www.sleepfoundation.org/children-and-sleep/how-blue-light-affects-kids-sleep

Teague, K. (2019, May 21). *Google tracks your purchases. Here's how to see what Gmail knows.* CNET. https://www.cnet.com/tech/mobile/google-tracks-your-purchases-heres-how-to-see-what-gmail-knows/

Thiefels, J. (2019, March 27). *Understanding Your Digital Footprint.* Net Nanny. https://www.netnanny.com/blog/what-every-teen-needs-to-know-about-their-digital-footprint/

Tween and teen health. (2022, February 26). Mayo Clinic. https://www.mayoclinic.org/healthy-lifestyle/tween-and-teen-health/in-depth/teens-and-social-media-use/art-20474437

Waltower, S. (2023, October 23). *How much time do Americans spend online and texting?* Business News Daily. https://www.businessnewsdaily.com/4718-weekly-online-social-media-time.html

Weir, K. (2023, September 1). *Social media brings benefits and risks to teens. Here's how psychology can help identify a path forward.* American Psychological Association. https://www.apa.org/monitor/2023/09/protecting-teens-on-social-media

Why your teen needs to worry about blue light. (n.d.). Vision Source. https://www.mccormickvision.com/eyecare/why-your-teen-needs-to-worry-about-blue-light/

Image References

Geralt. (2017, March 22). *Artificial intelligence, robot, ai* [image]. Pixabay.https://pixabay.com/photos/artificial-intelligence-robot-ai-2167835/

Kaboompics. (2015, May 30). *Lipstick, lipgloss* [image]. Pixabay. https://pixabay.com/photos/lipstick-lipgloss-lip-gloss-lips-791761/

Koch, A. (2022, January 28). *Student, man, desperate* [image]. Pixabay. https://pixabay.com/photos/student-man-desperate-depression-6976999/

Leninscape. (2017, April 12). *Yoga, woman, nature* [image]. Pixabay.https://pixabay.com/photos/yoga-woman-lake-outdoors-2176668/

Pexels. (2016, November 20). *Woman, Smartphone, Technology* [image]. Pixabay. https://pixabay.com/photos/woman-smartphone-technology-1847044/

Sammmie. (2016, March 17). *Friends, together, hugs* [image]. Pixabay. https://pixabay.com/photos/friends-together-hugs-back-view-1262152/

Sankowski, D. (2015, November 9). *Iphone, 6s, Plus* [image]. Pixabay.https://pixabay.com/photos/iphone-6s-plus-iwatch-apple-white-1032783/

Sasint. (2016, November 17). *Tired, young, laptop* [image]. Pixabay. https://pixabay.com/photos/tired-young-laptop-beautiful-1822678/

Stock Snap. (2015, September 3). *Shibuya crossing, Tokyo, Japan* [image]. Pixabay. https://pixabay.com/photos/shibuya-crossing-tokyo-japan-asia-923000/

Visual Worker. (2015, August 10). *Girl, t-shirt* [image]. Pixabay. https://pixabay.com/photos/girl-black-t-shirt-female-woman-882336/